Developmental &Functional Hand Grasps

Sandra J. Edwards, MA, OTR, FAOTA
Occupational Therapy Department
Western Michigan University
Kalamazoo, Michigan

Donna J. Buckland, MS, OTR
The Belle Center
St. Louis, Missouri

Jenna D. McCoy-Powlen, MS, OTR
Pasadena, California

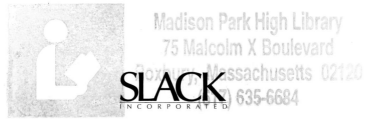

SLACK
INCORPORATED

An innovative information, education and management company
6900 Grove Road • Thorofare, NJ 08086

The procedures and practices described in this book should be implemented in a manner consistent with the professional standards set for the circumstances that apply in each specific situation. Every effort has been made to confirm the accuracy of the information presented and to correctly relate generally accepted practices. The author, editor, and publisher cannot accept responsibility for errors or exclusions or for the outcome of the application of the material presented herein. There is no expressed or implied warranty of this book or information imparted by it.

The work SLACK publishes is peer reviewed. Prior to publication, recognized leaders in the field, educators, and clinicians provide important feedback on the concepts and content that we publish. We welcome feedback on this work.

Edwards, Sandra J.
   Developmental and functional hand grasps / Sandra J. Edwards, Donna J. Buckland, Jenna D. McCoy-Powlen.
      p. ; cm.
   Includes bibliographical references and index.
   ISBN 1-55642-544-9 (alk. paper)
   1. Hand--Abnormalities--Diagnosis. 2. Disability evaluation. [DNLM: 1. Hand Strength--physiology. WE 830 E26d 2002] I.
      Buckland, Donna J. II. McCoy-Powlen, Jenna D. III. Title.
   RD778 .E35 2002
   617.5'750754--dc21   2002010249

Printed in the United States of America.

Published by: SLACK Incorporated
                  6900 Grove Road
                  Thorofare, NJ 08086 USA
                  Telephone: 856-848-1000
                  Fax: 856-853-5991
                  www.slackbooks.com

Last digit is print number: 10 9 8 7 6 5 4 3 2 1

CONTENTS

ACKNOWLEDGMENTS

We who choose to write books that include a lot of science, facts, photographs, and illustrations are very much in debt to the many people who have been so very kind and supportive to us. We have read others' articles, reviewed their pictures and sketches, and taken many ideas from their hard work. It is in the references that we acknowledge them in some respectable way. A lot of our information was derived from conversations, bits and pieces of things we've read or heard, and wonderful ideas we've read "somewhere." To all of those people we are grateful.

We are happy to express our gratitude, and acknowledge the many people who have assisted us in such important and meaningful ways. For the review of the content of the book we would like to thank Cindy Vinnex, OTR, CHT; Nancy Krolikowski, MS, OTR, CHT; Mary Ann Bush, MA, OTR, FAOTA; Natalie Turner, OTR; Kristen Chelgren; Stephanie Young; and Jennifer LeRoy. For their assistance and support we would like to thank the faculty at Western Michigan University's Occupational Therapy Department. For their contribution to the photographs we would like to thank graphic artists Lesli Banek and Christina Reid.

For allowing us to photograph their hands, we would like to thank Al Garcia, Mike and Michi Amemiya, Adrian Barkley, Victor Rumph, Lindsey Ross, Taylor Gamble, Kayleigh Gamble, Logan Downey, Nathan Downey, Adam Zink, Kristina Powlen, Jack and Susan McCoy, Cami McCoy, Edith and Wendell McCoy, and Craig Powlen.

For patience and moral support, we would like to thank Al Garcia; John and Rick Garcia; Jeanette Edwards; Craig Powlen; Jack and Susan McCoy; Cami McCoy; Edith and Wendell McCoy; Cara Gamble; Wilma, Gerald, and Julia Buckland; and Larry Gallen.

For the support of editors and staff at SLACK Incorporated, we would like to thank Amy McShane, John Bond, and Lauren Plummer.

INTRODUCTION

It is our hope that after reading our book you will share, as we do, a keener and more in-depth appreciation of the hand and its ability to grasp. Where would we be without our hands? This is a foreboding question. These remarkable parts of our anatomy are gifts that all of us use to fulfill the daily occupations of our lives and attain our dreams. We usually take them for granted. But underneath the skin is an incredible architecture and highly tuned nerve and muscle systems that give us a virtuosity of choreographed movements that provide manual dexterity, which gives us the ability to grasp objects. Anthropologists theorize that some of these grasps are millions of years old and others only thousands of years old. We use several different grasps in a minute without a sound or expense, but with remarkable grace. Bell (1834) portrayed a profound lesson that, "no serious account of human life can ignore the central importance of the human hand" (cited by Wilson, 1998, p. 7).

This book focuses on one aspect of the typical hand—its grasp. We had to consider what turned out to be a very difficult question: where exactly does the hand and its grasp begin? Clearly it is part of the bigger aspect of the body, encompassing the brain, posture, cognition, perception, and all the other systems in the body, directly or indirectly. To fulfill our mission of concisely and accurately presenting hand grasps, we agonizingly set firm boundaries as to what we would include in this book. Therefore, the text may mention—but does not cover—theory, treatment, or pathology of the hand. Other accompanying topics that are mentioned are posture, reach, approach, finger placement, release, and in-hand manipulation.

In clinical practice, it is important to identify and communicate to other professionals the grasp a client is using for a particular activity during an evaluation or treatment session. Whether working with an infant learning to grasp and manipulate objects in his or her environment, a child learning handwriting, or an adult with a stroke or hand injury, documentation of grasp can be difficult, especially with the many varieties of terms and inconsistent definitions and portrayals of those terms. Research studies using grasp terms as a means of measure are difficult to compare and contrast because of these inconsistencies. The purpose of this text is to clarify the confusion, eliminate the discrepancies, and put definitive labels on grasps. This text provides researchers, physicians, therapists, teachers, and other health professionals with common terms about hand grasps that will benefit our professions, research, and clients.

To develop the text of this book, we completed a thorough, in-depth review of the literature ranging from 1831 to 2002. Because of the discrepancies in terms and categories encountered in the literature, it was necessary to make decisions about the selection of terms based on the pervasiveness of the term in question, which researchers and authors used the term, and the potential confusion of the term with another or with its definition. To do this, we used our clinical and academic experience, and also consulted with an orthopedic surgeon, certified hand therapists, school-based therapists, academicians, and scholars. To best portray to the reader these descriptions of and neuromusculoskeletal components of each grasp, we consulted with a photographer, technicians, and an artist. We have organized and analyzed an enormous amount of highly complex information and condensed it into a usable size while striving for a concise, efficient, and clear format.

The photographs were taken of each grasp to give an accurate visual portrayal of the hand as well as to show the grasp in the context of functional activities. The hands that appear in the text are ones belonging to infants and adults between the ages of 2 weeks and 80 years with no pathology. The photographs of people's hands and activities represent a broad diversity of cultures from many regions of the world. Illustrations were designed to portray important anatomical features pertinent to grasp and to the understanding of the terms and definitions used throughout the text.

The content is organized as follows:

Chapter One, How to Observe and Examine the Hand for Grasp, is a compilation of information by physicians, certified hand therapists, and clinicians that give guidelines for observing the hand. Information about taking history, observing the general appearance, skin, dermatoglyphics, and nails is discussed. Information that is used to assess the circulation, musculoskeletal, sensory, and neurological integrity is discussed and related to clinical application relevant to hand grasps.

Chapter Two, Pictorial View of the Structure of the Hand as Related to Grasp, is a series of labeled illustrations that provide a pictorial view of the structure of the hand. This information was designed to identify the bones, joints, nerves, muscles, web spaces, ligaments, and arches of the hand that are discussed throughout the book.

Chapter Three, Reflexive Behaviors that Influence Grasp, discusses the impact of infant reflexes on the acquisition of grasp. Photographs of the response to the stimuli as well as descriptions and tables of the reflexes are the formats used to present this complicated information. A narrative summary of the interrelationship of these reflexes and their contribution to the development of grasp is included because of the relevance to evaluation and treatment of hand grasps.

Chapter Four, Development of Grasp, is a pictorial summary of the developmental stages of hand grasps. A narrative includes a referenced description, the developmental age at which each grasp is expected to emerge, and a very clinically useful discussion of developmental advancements. Also included in this chapter are tables to further clarify the age and titles used by numerous researchers who referenced each developmental grasp.

Chapter Five, Grasps for Handwriting, covers 12 pencil grasps used for handwriting that are most commonly observed in clinical practice, including school-based settings. The introduction to this chapter contains extensive pertinent information about these grasps and defines the development of the primitive, transitional, and mature pencil grasps. These photographs of children's and adults' pencil grasps represent clear and accurate detailed positions of the arm, wrist, fingers, and thumb. Each photograph is accompanied by a description carefully explaining each grasp.

Chapter Six, Functional Hand Grasps, is a collection of grasps commonly used by the adult or child to perform occupational tasks involved in daily living. A researched description accompanies each photograph. The grasps are divided into groups: power, precision, combined power/precision, miscellaneous, and nonprehensile movements, and are then arranged alphabetically within these divisions. A brief overview of muscles is given, along with interesting information and functional uses.

We envision all these chapters as being useful both clinically and academically. Researchers can also use them with confidence. We invite you to learn and enjoy your own hands and the hands of those around you as they all tell our life stories.

Sandra J. Edwards, MA, OTR, FAOTA
Donna J. Buckland, MS, OTR
Jenna D. McCoy-Powlen, MS, OTR

CHAPTER ONE

How to Observe and Examine the Hand for Grasp

This chapter provides guidelines for the important task of clinically examining the hand in relation to grasp. Clinical exam, according to Thomine (1981), is the most significant source of information. Radiological, electrical, and thermographic exams supply augmentative information. It is only by using the professional's observation and interview from the clinical exam that the state of the skin, joints, muscles, tendons, and nerves can be properly assessed. The same applies to the assessment of functional grasp used in activities of daily living.

It is suggested that the initial evaluation include a deductive as well as an inductive approach to select assessments. The deductive (or "top down") approach facilitates a better understanding of the person and how the concern for the hand grasp is affecting that individual's life. Trombly (1995b) reports that an understanding of life roles is of primary importance when beginning the evaluation process. Interview is an effective method to obtain this information. The inductive reasoning (or "bottom up") approach provides important clinical detail for intervention strategies, which includes more of the physical components related to grasp.

As stated in the book's introduction, the hand grasp is a complex component of a highly involved process performed by the body. The act of grasping is not confined to the hand or even the arm, but is dependent on the entire body for the stability necessary for successful prehension. In fact, the strength and stability of the trunk and the upper extremity in question should be considered because distal symptoms may be caused by proximal problems (Cooper, 2002). Because an in-depth discussion on proximal strength and stability is beyond the scope of this book, the following chapter focuses on the observation and assessment of the hand and the components necessary to accomplish grasp.

HISTORY AND PRESENT CONDITION

Functional History

- Determine the functional tasks that are important to the individual's life roles. This information will assist the clinician in determining which grasps are most significant in the individual's life.
- Document the occupational history, psychosocial history, education, and the individual's goals for treatment.

Medical History

- Via interview, document the presenting concern, onset, past injuries, medical condition, gender, age, hand dominance, and current functions of the hand.

- Obtain information about past therapy, the person's response to it, and their understanding of the therapy process. This information assists the clinician in knowing whether the person has educational and/or psychological needs.

Document General Appearance

- Before administering a standardized functional assessment, it is beneficial to observe the person in the context of doing meaningful activity (Duff, Shumway-Cook, & Woollacott, 2001).
- Observe the general appearance of the limb by assessing the posture and position in which the hand is being held. The condition of the contralateral hand should also be noted.
- Observe both the affected and unaffected hand at rest and note how the hand is being held while the individual is walking and sitting.

ASSESSMENT OF PAIN

- Assess subjective pain using interview, history, questionnaire, body diagrams, or pain rating scales. Pain restricts movement, decreasing active range of motion and causing loss of the muscle strength that is necessary for grasp. Pain may determine which grasps are used and the strength of those grasps.
- Cooper (2002) states that pain needs to be carefully assessed to identify whether it is chronic or acute. Acute pain serves to protect; chronic pain may originate from myofascial pain signaling irritation in fascia, muscle, tendon, or ligament.
- Determine location of the pain, frequency, intervals, and if present during rest or only during movement.

EXAMINATION OF SKIN COVERING, CREASES, DERMATOGLYPHICS, AND NAILS

Assessing the features of the skin and nails is an important part of looking at the hand as it can yield important clues to the function of the hand.

I. The **skin** is a vital organ that not only protects the underlying structures of the hand, but houses many minute structures that are essential to a successful grasp.

    A. Document general appearance: Examine the appearance of the skin for atrophy by noting any shiny appearance or thinness. In addition, observe for wrinkles, color, texture, sweat, hair patterns, temperature (test by moving distal to proximal for differences), ulcers, gangrene, and swelling. Note the presence of any blisters, as these may indicate injurious hand use due to sensory loss (Cooper, 2002). Observe for fragile skin in the older person, in individuals with diabetes, or in those who have taken steroids for a prolonged period.

    B. Scars: Assess the hand for abnormal thickness, such as scars or calluses.

        i. Scars need to be carefully examined to determine location, length, width, and height. Note any adherence of skin and tendon that may restrict movement (Cooper, 2002).

        ii. Location of scars: Note whether a scar crosses any joints and if that scar restricts the motion of the joint (Cooper, 2002).

            a. Longitudinal palmar scars cross the flexion creases and are the most commonly seen (Thomine, 1981).

                1. Contractures of these scars interfere with finger extension and, therefore, proper finger placement for grasp.

                2. Finger flexion may also be affected, which interferes with many grasps.

            b. Scars within the web spaces of the fingers and thumb are also commonly seen.

                1. Contractures of these scars can invade the palmar interdigital system and restrict the metacarpophalangeal (MCP) joints. The restriction of these joints may result in the

inability to provide stabilization in the MCP flexion used in distal precision grasps, such as the *three jaw chuck*.

    2. Web space scars may also limit the ability to isolate the MCP flexion to any one joint. This would interfere with grasps that require extension of one MCP joint and flexion of an adjacent MCP joint, such as a *diagonal volar grasp*.

    3. These scars may also limit the amount of finger abduction, which would compromise the ability to grasp large objects using the *disc grasp*.

II. **Creases** of the hand and wrist include digital, opposition, palmar, and wrist creases.

    A. Assess for the presence of middle and distal wrist creases, proximal and distal palmar creases, as well as opposition and finger flexion creases.

    B. These creases are in close proximity to, but not always directly over, the joints of the hand and are the areas where the hand is able to move. These creases are important landmarks for splinting purposes (Duncan, 1989). They identify the axis of motion for the corresponding joint (Callinan, 2002).

    C. Creases are an important part of the architecture of the hand, allowing flexion and cupping of the hand, such as in the *lumbrical grasp* and the *spherical grasp*, respectively.

    D. Absence of these creases can be observed in individuals with genetic syndromes, such as Turner's or Down syndrome. A lack of creases inhibits cupping of grasp and restricts the movement of the arches in the hand. This inhibition is detrimental to any grasp that needs to accommodate the size and shape of an object.

III. **Dermatoglyphics** of the hand include the fingerprints and their components. Each person has unique patterns of swirls and loops on the pads of their fingers.

    A. The ridges of the fingerprints contain papillary glands that secrete sweat, providing friction during grasping. This is important for both power and precision grasps in that objects held or secured by the pads of the fingers are held in place, in part, by the friction of the dermatoglyphics.

    B. The moisture secreted by the sweat glands within the dermatoglyphics also helps objects stick to the pads of the fingers. This can be observed while turning the pages of a book using the *pad to pad grasp* or opening a jar using the *opposed palmar grasp*.

    C. The loss of these ridges greatly affects grasp and manipulation. The friction normally provided by these ridges is minimized. This makes daily activities, such as picking up coins and making change with paper bills, very difficult.

    D. Certain professionals, such as hairdressers, can lose these dermatoglyphic features because they repeatedly expose their hands to chemicals that literally wear away their fingerprints.

IV. **Nail changes** can affect grasp because the nail matrix supports the pulp or fat pads of the fingertips.

    A. Nails can be observed for thickness, thinness, atrophy, or loss.

    B. Nail changes can affect grasp because the nail matrix supports the pulp or fat pads of the fingertips. Integrity of the thumb and finger pulps are important in grasps in that this fat pad helps to cushion the object on the fingertips and thumb, improving the stability of the object being grasped.

    C. Loss of or atrophic changes in the nails may affect grasp by affecting the support of the finger pads, whose integrity are crucial to most grasps.

    D. Thick nails can be a symptom for a genetic anomaly, such as Turner's syndrome.

EXAMINATION OF CIRCULATION

Proper circulation of blood through the radial and ulnar arteries and circulation of lymphatic fluid is important for optimal use of the hand.

I. **Vascular system:** A compromise in the vascular system can cause ischemia, which is hypoxia of the tissues as a result of inadequate blood flow.

    A. Ischemia may result in a compromise of skin integrity, pain, and weakness, all of which affect the optimal function of the hand and its grasp.

    B. Assessment of vascular compromise.

        i. Examine the color of the hand and nails: Vascular compromise is strongly suspected when cyanosis, erythema, gangrene, or a grayish color is observed (Cooper, 2002).

ii. Check for pulses and note the temperature of the extremity.

iii. Assess circulation by pressing the nail beds until they turn white. Then release the pressure, noting when color returns (should be within two seconds of release). Compare the results with the uninvolved hand or digits (Cooper, 2002). This is indicative of the adequacy of blood flow to the fingertips.

iv. Allen's test checks the patency of the radial and ulnar arteries. This test is done by placing pressure on the radial or ulnar arteries at the wrist and having the person repeatedly make a fist. The person opens the hand and the pressure to the artery is released; observe the return of blood to hand (Van Deusen & Brunt, 1997).

II. **Lymphatic system:** A compromise in the lymphatic system may result in edema, which is excess fluids present within body tissues.

A. Assessment of edema: Circumference and volumetric measurements estimate the amount of edema present in tissues and can be used before and after treatment to objectively analyze size changes in the hand.

i. Circumference of the forearm is used to assist with measuring the amount of edema in the hand or forearm. Measure the circumference of the forearm and the wrist and compare to the opposite arm measured at same point.

ii. Volumetric measurement measures the amount of edema in the hand or arm. This is accomplished by immersing the affected extremity into a marked container and measuring the amount of water that is displaced. This value is then compared to the amount of water displaced when the uninvolved extremity is immersed.

B. Excessive edema can interfere with hand function because of the restricted range of motion in the finger and thumb joints, resulting in the loss of function and stiffness of the hand.

EXAMINATION OF LIGAMENTS AND MUSCLES

Ligaments and muscles serve many important purposes, including maintaining joint stability and movement (Lockhart, Hamilton, & Fyfe, 1959).

I. **Ligaments** play an important role in stabilizing joints. Without the joint stability provided by the ligaments, prehension would be impossible.

A. Major Types of Ligaments

i. Radiocarpal/Ulnocarpal Ligaments

a. Location: Between radius and carpal bones and ulna and carpal bones. These ligaments are located in the area of the distal wrist crease and the base of the hand.

b. Function: Connects the radius to the carpal bones and the ulna to the carpal bones. Provides carpal stability during grasp and permits range of motion of the wrist.

ii. Intercapsular and Intracapsular Ligaments

a. Location: On the surface of and in between the carpal bones located at the base of the palm.

b. Function: Connects the carpal bones to each other. Provides carpal stability and permits range of motion of the wrist.

iii. Carpometacarpal Ligaments (Palmar and Dorsal)

a. Location: Located between the carpal and metacarpal bones. Forms the carpometacarpal (CMC) joints at the base of the palm.

b. Function: Connects the carpal bones to the metacarpal bones. Provides stability for the wrist and metacarpals and permits range of motion at these CMC joints.

iv. Metacarpal Ligaments (Dorsal, Palmar, Deep Transverse)

a. Location: Connects the metacarpal bones to each other between the anterior aspects of the proximal phalanges and between the necks of metacarpals, which are located near the web spaces between the fingers.

b. Function: Assists with reinforcing flexor muscles, provides stability to the hand for grasp.

        v. Collateral Ligaments (Cord, Accessory, Palmar Fibro-Cartilaginous Plate)

           a. Location: Connects the metacarpals bones to the phalangeal bones, creating the MCP joints. Also connects the phalangeal bones together to support the interphalangeal (IP) joints of the fingers and thumb.

           b. Function: Oblique configuration of these ligaments provides lateral stability and assists the extensor muscles with reinforcing finger and thumb joints (Strickland, 1995), which increases the mechanical advantage for flexor tendons.

      vi. Distal Flexor Sheath (Annular and Cruciate Pulleys)

           a. Location: Volar side of the hand beginning at the metacarpal heads and moving to the distal phalanges.

           b. Function: These pulleys maintain proper alignment of the tendons with the axis of the digits, preventing anterior-posterior and lateral shifts (University of Kansas Medical Center, 1997).

  B. To assess ligament stability, shift different bone structures and note the mobility in each joint.

     i. Collateral ligaments: These ligaments provide lateral stability to the joint. To assess these, gently resist these joints from the lateral side of the finger on the horizontal plane to determine stability and/or laxity.

    ii. Volar ligaments: These ligaments prevent hyperextension of the joints. To assess these, gently apply resistance to the joint to determine its level of laxity in extension. As the individual actively opens and closes his or her hand, observe for smoothness and continuity of movement.

   iii. Contralateral hand: Also assess the unaffected side as different people have varying levels of mobility in their joints.

II. **Muscles:** A certain level of strength and stability are necessary to grasp. This level varies, depending on the activity to be performed and the size of the object to be held.

  A. Testing Muscle Strength

     i. Perform a manual muscle test of fingers, thumb, wrist, and arm.

    ii. Strength of power grasps can be measured using a dynamometer for adults or a Martin Vigorimeter (Elmed Inc., Addison, IL, 312-543-2792) for children or individuals with arthritis (Link, Lukens, & Bush, 1995). Strength of pinch grasp can be measured by using a pinch meter.

  B. Muscle Tone: Examine the muscle tone by observing for hypotonicity (low tone) or hypertonicity (increased tone), as both will affect grasping and contribute to fatigue and poor coordination.

     i. Increased tone will inhibit the isolation of individual fingers for precision grasps.

    ii. Flaccid tone will compromise stability in precision grasps and the strength of power grasps.

  C. Movement: Note the smoothness, control, and accuracy of the movement, as well as the range of motion in the joints of the hands.

EXAMINATION OF BONES, JOINTS, AND ARCHES

These anatomical components of the hand are the underlying structures upon which the soft tissues function.

I. **Bones:** Our hands are precisely balanced to allow each bone to move in planes that enable us to perform intricate movements and manipulations. Alteration in the morphology of these precisely formed bones can interrupt that balance, resulting in difficulty grasping and performing functional tasks.

  A. Examine the shape and structure or morphology.

     i. Thickness of bones.

    ii. Bony landmarks.

   iii. Curvature of phalanges. This is sometimes seen in the little finger, resulting in difficulty opposing the thumb with the hypothenar eminence.

  B. Examine the length of fingers and thumb and width of palm.

     i. Weiss and Flatt (1971) found that the length of the finger is positively correlated with pinch strength.

    ii. Link et al. (1995) found that hand width was positively correlated with grip strength.

        iii. Some genetic syndromes like Down syndrome cause the person to have shorter phalanges in the fingers and thumbs. This may cause problems with opposition and prehension and ultimately result in difficulty with precision grasps, such as the *neat pincer grasp*.

II. **Joints:** There is no joint articulation that is in itself an isolated mechanical entity. Instead, each articulation is a component of a group arranged in kinetic chains (Benbow, 1995).

    A. Evaluate passive and active range of motion of wrist, thumb, and fingers.

    B. Assess functional range of motion by observing the individual.

        i. Open and close the hand.

        ii. Oppose the thenar and hypothenar eminences.

        iii. Oppose the thumb.

    C. Note any articular swelling and effusion (which is the escape of any fluid such as pus, blood, or serum).

III. **Arches** are musculoskeletal structures that provide flattening and cupping of the hand (Henderson & Pehoski, 1995) and help to enable a strong functional grasp. The flattening and cupping of the palm allow the hand to grasp objects of varying size, and are therefore necessary for optimal hand function. There are four main structural arches. One is rigid (transverse carpal arch) and the others are mobile (transverse metacarpal arch, longitudinal arch [Duncan, 1989] , and opposition arch [Benbow, 2002]).

    A. Transverse arches: Observe the transverse arches located across the heel of the hand and the metacarpal pads; they provide curvature of the hand for grasping objects such as in the *diagonal volar* and *hammer grasps*.

        i. Transverse Carpal Arch

            a. Location: The distal carpal bones provide its structure.

            b. Function: This structure is a stable point that allows a pivot for the interplay of wrist and middle finger bones (Coppard & Lohman, 1996). The transverse carpal ligament and the carpal bones contained in this arch are the passage for the extrinsic finger flexors and form the carpal tunnel. This ligament provides a mechanical feature to the finger extrinsic tendons that serves as a pulley (Coppard & Lohman, 1996). This arch can be seen while using a *spherical grasp*.

        ii. Transverse Metacarpal Arch

            a. Location: This arch is formed slightly below the MCP joint.

            b. Function: It is known as the flexible arch (Coppard & Lohman, 1996) in that this arch deepens with motion. This movement is necessary for optimal hand function (Duncan, 1989). Ulnar denervation flattens the ulnar portion of this arch, adversely affecting grasp (Cooper, 2002). A flattened arch of the palm can weaken the grasp of large objects (Tubiana, Thomine, & Mackin, 1996). This arch can be seen while using a *ventral grasp*.

        iii. Longitudinal Arch

            a. Location: This arch consists of the carpal bones, metacarpals, and phalanges.

            b. Function: The mobility of the first, fourth, and fifth MCP joints allow these joints to move in relationship to the shape and size of the object in the palm. The relative stability of the second and third fingers and radial palm allows grasping and holding of objects (Duncan, 1989). The arch is formed by the carpals, metacarpals, and phalanges of each finger and works in concert with the muscles to form the long arch that allows cupping of the hand for grasp. The action of this arch can be seen when using a *cylindrical grasp* (Boehme, 1988).

        iv. Opposition or Diagonal Arches

            a. Location: Consists of the metacarpal as well as the proximal and distal phalanxes of the thumb as it opposes the fingers (Benbow, 2002).

            b. Function: These "arches are active while holding, stabilizing, and directing tools as an extension of the hand" (Benbow, 1999, pg. 22). The action of this arch can be seen when using a *diagonal volar grasp*.

EXAMINATION OF SENSORY DISCRIMINATION AND SENSORY POSITION

Sensation is necessary for successful grasp and prehension. Intact sensation enables the hand to precisely fit around the object to be grasped, while providing information such as position, dimension, weight, and force needed to secure the object. If sensation is compromised, it becomes necessary to rely on other sensations such as vision, which requires greater cognitive attention. As a result, prehension is clumsy and objects are often crushed in the hands or dropped (Nakada & Uchida, 1997).

I. **Sensory discrimination tests** are valid predictors of hand function (Bell-Krotoski, Weinstein, & Weinstein, 1993; Dellon & Kallman, 1983; Gordon & Duff, 1999). Cooper (2002) states that the Semmes-Weinstein monofilaments (Sammons Preston, Bolingbrook, IL, 1-800-323-5547) and the static two-point discrimination tests are the most widely used sensibility tests in hand therapy.

   A. Touch pressure sensitivity: Semmes-Weinstein monofilaments are a standardized assessment using a set of nylon monofilaments of various diameters that examine a person's threshold of touch perception.

      i. To test, have the individual indicate whether he or she perceives touch when a monofilament is applied to various parts of the hand (with vision occluded).

      ii. This sensitivity to touch pressure may influence grasp, in that this sensation helps us to determine the force needed to be applied to the object that is to be grasped.

   B. Static two-point discrimination measures how far apart two static tactile stimuli have to be on a given body part to be perceived as two separate stimuli.

      i. To test, use calipers to apply two simultaneous tactile stimulations to various parts of the hand, having the individual indicate whether one or two stimuli are perceived. Note the distance between the stimuli that is necessary for the perception of two separate stimuli.

      ii. The inability to discriminate within normal range can significantly affect the ability to grasp and manipulate objects during activities of daily living.

II. **Sensory position:** Proprioception is the perception of the position of body parts, which is assessed without vision. Stereognosis is the ability to recognize objects with vision occluded while relying on the senses of touch and proprioception.

   A. Proprioception

      i. To test, move the limb and ask the person to reproduce the movement in the contralateral hand or identify if the body part is "up" or "down."

      ii. Proprioception is important in power grasps, but is especially important in precision grasps. The reason for this is that when grasping a very small object using a precision grasp, like the *tip pinch*, it is often not possible to fully visualize the object being grasped. As a result, proprioceptive and other sensory feedback is necessary for a successful grasp.

   B. Stereognosis

      i. To test, allow the person to manipulate common objects in the environment (such as coins, keys, comb, etc.) and identify the object with vision occluded, taking into consideration the individual's cultural background and the probable familiarity with the presented objects.

      ii. Stereognosis is important to grasp, in that without the ability to recognize an object by touch it is necessary to continually depend on vision to manipulate objects in the environment. This requires greater cognitive attention and affects fluency of manipulation.

EXAMINATION OF THE RADIAL NERVE

The radial nerve innervates muscles that extend the wrist and fingers (Brandenberg, Hawkins, & Quick, 1999). The radial nerve also helps to enable extension and abduction of the thumb (Brandenberg et al., 1999). The radial nerve innervates the dorsal aspect of the radial side of the hand (Cooper, 2002).

I. **Motor Function**

   A. The Intact Radial Nerve

      i. Effects on the thumb: The radial nerve assists with the abduction (abductor pollicis longus) and extension (extensor pollicis brevis) (Strickland, 1995) of the thumb that opens the web space between the thumb and the index finger. The opening of the web space allows the hand to grasp objects of multiple sizes (Tubiana et al., 1996). These movements are also important components in thumb opposition, which is a crucial part of most grasps.

    ii. Effects on digits 2 through 5: An intact radial nerve is important for grasping, in that it assists with the extension of the fingers (extensor indicis, extensor digitorum, and extensor digiti minimi) (Reed, 1991) into proper finger placement for grasping large objects.

    iii. Effects on wrist: The radial nerve innervates some of the muscles that allow extension and ulnar deviation of the wrist (extensor carpi ulnaris), both of which enhance the power of the grasp. This nerve also enables the function of the extensor carpi radialis longus and brevis, which extends and radially deviates the wrist (Strickland, 1995). The extension of the wrist makes tenodesis possible (Cooper, 2002).

  B. The Injured Radial Nerve

    i. Effects on the thumb: An injured radial nerve will compromise the ability to extend and abduct the thumb. This will also disrupt manipulation skills because the ability to open the web space is essential for grasping large objects (Tubiana et al., 1996). The loss of this innervation compromises these movements of the thumb that are important for power grasps, such as the *reverse transverse palmar* and the *oblique palmer grasp*, as well as precision grasps, such as a *disc grasp*.

    ii. Effects on digits 2 through 5: The inability to extend the fingers makes precise finger placement for grasping difficult. Even grasping small objects requires some amount of finger extension to open the hand to accommodate the object. If the distal phalanges cannot fully extend, the grasp of large objects will be compromised (Tubiana et al., 1996), such as with a *spherical grasp*.

    iii. Effects on wrist: Because the injured radial nerve cannot properly extend the wrist, the individual's ability to grasp objects or make a fist is compromised due to "wrist drop," which interferes with the action of the flexor muscles. Also, as a result of the inability to extend the wrist, tenodesis is lost. This nerve is critical to a person who has experienced a spinal cord injury due to the importance of the tenodesis action (Cooper, 2002).

II. **Sensory Component of Radial Nerve**

  A. The intact radial nerve innervates the dorsal aspect of the radial portion of the hand (Cooper, 2002).

  B. The injured radial nerve does not greatly affect prehension, as compared to the loss of the sensation to the palmar side of the hand (Cooper, 2002).

III. **To test the radial nerve,** ask the individual to hold the hands together at the base of the palms with extended fingers, forming a "V" shape, or have the individual hold the hands in a prayer position; if the hands and fingers cannot extend to assume these positions, then the radial nerve may be impaired.

EXAMINATION OF THE MEDIAN NERVE

The median nerve innervates some of the intrinsic flexors of the digits on the radial side of the hand, as well as the muscles that assist with thumb opposition, flexion, and abduction. The median nerve also innervates some of the extrinsic flexors of the wrist and fingers and the pronators in the forearm (Cooper, 2002). It also transmits sensation from some of the areas of the hand that are most used in grasping.

I. **Motor Function**

  A. The Intact Median Nerve

    i. Effects on the thumb: The median nerve assists with thumb opposition (opponens pollicis), abduction (abductor pollicis), and flexion (part of the flexor pollicis brevis) (Strickland, 1995). All of these movements are important in thumb opposition.

    ii. Effects on digits 2 through 5: The median nerve innervates various muscles that affect finger flexion. The flexion of the index and middle fingers depends on innervation of the lumbricals and the flexor digitorum profundus. The flexor digitorum profundus also enables distal interphalangeal (DIP) flexion of the index and sometimes the middle fingers (Tubiana et al., 1996). The flexion of all of the fingers depends on the innervation of the flexor digitorum superficialis (Cooper, 2002).

        iii. Effects on grasp: An intact median nerve is important in grasps that require flexion of the radial fingers. These grasps include many of both the precision and power grasps, such as the *tip pinch* and the *hammer grasp*. This nerve also helps enable thumb abduction, which is an important component of opposition and opens the web space for many grasps such as the *cylindrical grasp*, the *neat pincer grasp*, and the *dynamic tripod grasp*.

        iv. Effects on forearm position: The median nerve innervates the pronator quadratus and the pronator teres, which are vital for forearm pronation (Cooper, 2002).

        v. Effects on wrist: The median nerve innervates the flexor carpi radialis that assists with wrist flexion and radial deviation (Strickland, 1995). Radial deviation positions the hand for nonprehensile hand movements (such as playing piano) as well as for precision grasps.

  B. The Injured Median Nerve

        i. Effects on the thumb: Denervation of the median nerve compromises thumb abduction, opposition, and flexion. The thumb may rest in adduction and become contracted (Cooper, 2002). The impairment of these movements would greatly affect any grasp requiring thumb opposition, such as the *interdigital tripod grasp*, the *three jaw chuck*, or the *ring grasp*.

        ii. Effects on digits 2 through 5: The ability to flex the radial fingers would be lost with the paralysis of the median nerve. This movement is a major component in most grasps, including the *oblique palmar grasp* and the *pad to pad*.

        iii. Effects on grasp: The ability to abduct and oppose the thumb is imperative in most grasps, including handwriting grasps, and would be compromised with an injured median nerve. The DIP flexion of the thumb, index, and sometimes the middle fingers necessary to perform the *tip pinch* is lost with the paralysis of this nerve. Also, the loss of this movement decreases the strength of a power grasp (Tubiana et al., 1996), such as the *opposed palmar grasp*. When the median nerve is compressed, such as in carpal tunnel syndrome, the individual may experience weakness, numbness, tingling, and pain in the hand and wrist, all of which adversely affect grasp.

        iv. Effects on forearm position: Pronation for certain activities would become difficult, although substitution activities (e.g., accessory muscles and gravity) would assist with this movement (Hislop & Montgomery, 1995).

        v. Effects on wrist: The ability to radially deviate would be affected by the disruption of the median nerve.

II. Sensory Component of the Median Nerve

  A. The intact median nerve supplies sensation to the radial side of the volar aspect of the hand (Tubiana et al., 1996). This nerve is responsible for the innervation of the pads of the fingers and thumb that we depend on most for prehension.

  B. The injured median nerve greatly interferes with prehension because the area of innervation is so vital for grasps (Cooper, 2002).

III. To Assess the Median Nerve

  A. Ask the person to make a fist and observe the radial fingers, which will not flex if the median nerve is injured or paralyzed.

  B. Another way to assess the integrity of the median nerve is to have the individual touch the pad of the thumb to the tip of each finger, and then ask him or her to maintain a strong pinch with the thumb and index finger. If he or she can do both of these exercises, then the median nerve is likely intact (Brandenberg et al., 1999).

EXAMINATION OF THE ULNAR NERVE

This nerve supplies many of the muscles used for flexion of the hand as well as sensation to the fingers for power grasping (Tubiana et al., 1996). It also supplies the muscles active in ulnar deviation of the wrist, which is important for the strength of the power grasp. Additionally, this nerve innervates the intrinsic muscles in the palm, which are critical for grasp. This nerve transmits sensation from the ulnar side of the hand.

I. **Motor Nerves**

    A. The Intact Ulnar Nerve

        i. Effects on the thumb: The ulnar nerve innervates muscles that assist with thumb adduction (adductor pollicis) and flexion (part of the flexor pollicis brevis) (Strickland, 1995), both of which are important movements in thumb opposition. These muscles are also important in that they add strength to the grasp (Tubiana et al., 1996). The adduction and flexion of the thumb is important in grasps, such as the *lateral pinch*.

        ii. Effects on digits 2 through 5: The ulnar nerve innervates dorsal and volar interossei, helping to enable abduction of digits 2 through 4 and adduction of digits 2 through 5. Those same muscles assist other muscles with flexion of the MCP joints while allowing extension of the IP joints of the fingers, such as in the *lumbrical grasp*. The ulnar nerve innervates lumbricals of the ring and little finger to supplement flexion and extension in those digits (Strickland, 1995).

        iii. Specific effects on little finger: The ulnar nerve innervates muscles that abduct (abductor digiti minimi), flex (flexor digiti minimi), and allow opposition (opponens digiti minimi) of the little finger (Reed, 1991).

        iv. Effects on wrist: The ulnar nerve innervates the flexor carpi ulnaris that assists with wrist flexion and ulnar deviation (Strickland, 1995). Ulnar deviation increases the strength of grasp.

    B. The Injured Ulnar Nerve

        i. Effects on the thumb: The loss of strength of the intrinsic thumb flexor (deep head only) and adductor results not only in a weakened grasp, but compromises the ability to bring the thumb and first finger together in a stable and precise pinch.

        ii. Effects on digits 2 through 5: The loss of the action of the interossei would compromise the ability to adduct and abduct the fingers. This is an essential movement in adjusting the hand to the size of the object to be grasped. The loss of innervation of the lumbricals and the flexor digitorum profundus within the ulnar side of the hand would compromise the strength of the grasp. The inability to use the interossei (which assist with MCP joint flexion while allowing IP joint extension) would affect the ability to use the *lumbrical grasp*. The loss of the function of this nerve would also compromise the ability to fully flex the fingers for a *cylindrical grasp* or to flex the distal joints for *hook grasp* (Reed, 1991). The loss of the action of the ulnar nerve would also result in a "claw hand," which is an inability of the intrinsic muscles to balance the extrinsic flexors and extensors (Philips, 1995). The claw deformity will vary depending on the specific injury to the ulnar nerve.

        iii. Effects on little finger: The denervation of the muscles that enable flexion, abduction, and opposition of the little finger results not only in a loss of those particular movements (Cooper, 2002), but also a compromise in the stability of various grasps. For example, the flexion of the 4th and 5th digits are important for the stabilization of all of the mature and most of the transitional pencil grasps. This stabilization force, provided by the ulnar fingers, is an essential backdrop for the precise movements made by the radial fingers during handwriting and other functional activities requiring precision. For other grasps, the addition of the ulnar digits adds greater power and stability, as with the *palmar grasp* and *hammer grasp*.

        iv. Effects on wrist: The ability to ulnarly deviate would be affected by the disruption of this nerve and would compromise the strength of many power grasps.

II. **Sensory component of the ulnar nerve:** The ulnar nerve provide sensory feedback from the dorsal and volar sides of the ulnar digits (Cooper, 2002) and the ulnar aspect of the palm.

III. **To Assess the Ulnar Nerve**

    A. Observe the use of the little finger; abduction indicates weak palmar interossei and unbalanced action of the long extensor tendon.

    B. To test the ulnar nerve, ask the person to clasp their fingers together; if the ring and little finger remain extended, this may indicate an impairment of this nerve.

    C. Another test of the ulnar nerve is to observe the function of the thumb adductor muscle. To do this, ask the individual to hold a piece of paper tightly between the adducted thumb and the index finger. If the paper is held tightly by thumb adduction and with no substitution of flexion of the thumb's IP joint, then the ulnar nerve is intact. If the thumb adductor muscle is weak, then the person will flex the IP joint of the thumb to compensate and this is called Froment's sign (Van Deusen & Brunt, 1997).

CHAPTER TWO

PICTORIAL VIEW OF THE STRUCTURE OF THE HAND AS RELATED TO GRASP

This chapter is designed to graphically present the essentials of the musculoskeletal anatomy that are pertinent to the following discussions of grasps. Included are:

1. Surface Anatomy of the Wrist and Hand
   - Dorsal View (Figure 2-1)
   - Volar View (Figure 2-2)
2. Positions of the Thumb (as depicted by Pact, Sirotkin-Roses, & Beatus, 1984)
   - Abduction (Figure 2-3)
   - Adduction (Figure 2-4)
   - Flexion (Figure 2-5)
   - Extension (Figure 2-6)
   - Opposition (Figure 2-7)
3. Bones of the Right Wrist and Hand
   - Dorsal View (Figure 2-8)
   - Volar View (Figure 2-9)
4. Ligaments of the Wrist
   - Dorsal View (Figure 2-10)
   - Volar View (Figure 2-11)
5. Ligaments of the Digital Joints (Figure 2-12A)
6. Digital Flexor Sheath (Figure 2-12B)
7. Intrinsic Muscles of the Thumb
   - Abductor Pollicis Brevis, Flexor Pollicis Brevis, and Opponens Pollicis (Figure 2-13)
   - Adductor Pollicis, Oblique, and Transverse Heads (Figure 2-14)

8. Intrinsic Muscles of the Palm of the Hand
   - Lumbricals (Figure 2-15)
   - Dorsal Interossei (Figure 2-16)
   - Volar Interossei (Figure 2-17)
   - Hypothenar Muscles: Abductor Digiti Minimi, Flexor Digiti Minimi Brevis, Opponens Digiti Minimi (Figure 2-18)
9. Superficial Extrinsic Muscles of the Forearm
   - Dorsal View (Figure 2-19)
   - Volar View (Figure 2-20)
10. Longitudinal and Transverse Arches of the Hand
    - Lateral View (Figure 2-21)
    - Palmar View (Figure 2-22)
11. Innervation of the Surface of the Hand for Sensation
    - Dorsal View (Figure 2-23)
    - Palmar View (Figure 2-24)

LANDMARKS ON THE SURFACE ANATOMY OF THE HAND

A. Styloid Process ....Located on the distal part of the ulna.

B. Styloid Process ....Located on the distal part of the radius.

C. Metacarpophalangeal ....Where the metacarpal bones connect with the proximal phalanx
Joints (MCP)   bones. The joints on the radial side of the hand are higher than the
ulnar side of the hand when the hand is fisted (Duncan, 1989).

D. Carpometacarpal Joint (CMC) ....Where the capitate bone connects with the metacarpal bone of the
thumb.

E. Proximal Interphalangeal ....Where the proximal phalanx connects with the middle phalanx.
Joints (PIP)   Located in the second through fifth digits, PIP and DIP joints of the
fingers are often referred to collectively as the IP joints.

F. Distal Interphalangeal...............................Where the middle phalanx connects with the distal phalanx.
Joints (DIP)   Located in the second through fifth digits, PIP and DIP joints of the
fingers are often referred to collectively as the IP joints.

G. Interphalangeal Joint (IP) ....Where the proximal phalanx of the thumb connects with the distal
phalanx of the thumb. This is the only IP joint located in the thumb.

H. Web Spaces ....The space between the digits. The space between the thumb and
index finger is the deepest and most flexible web space.

I. Distal Palmar Crease.................................Transverse flexion crease located proximal to the MCP joint of
the little finger and extends across the palm to a point between the
MCP joints of the index and middle fingers (Duncan, 1989).

J. Proximal Palmar Crease ....Transverse flexion crease located mid-palm, just proximal to the distal palmar crease. It extends across the palm from the hypothenar
eminence to the lateral side of the hand just above the opposition
crease.

K. Opposition Crease......................................Crease that surrounds the palmar boundary of the thenar eminence.

L. Finger Flexion Creases ....Creases located near the DIP, PIP, and MCP joints of the fingers, and
the IP and MCP joints of the thumb.

M. Distal Wrist Crease ....Extends across the wrist from the tubercle of the trapezium to the
pisiform bone, forming a line between the distal and proximal rows of
carpal bones (Duncan, 1989).

N. Middle Wrist Crease ....Transverse flexion crease located at the radiocarpal joint.

O. Thenar Eminence ....Bulge of muscles just proximal to the base of the thumb. Includes
three muscles: opponens pollicis, abductor pollicis brevis, and flexor
pollicis brevis.

P. Hypothenar Eminence ....Ulnar aspect of the palm that is the heel of the hand. Includes three
muscles: opponens digiti minimi, abductor digiti minimi, and flexor
digiti minimi brevis.

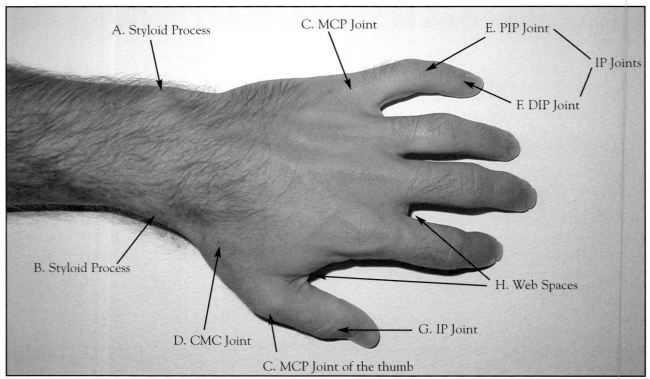

Figure 2-1. Surface anatomy of wrist and hand—dorsal view.

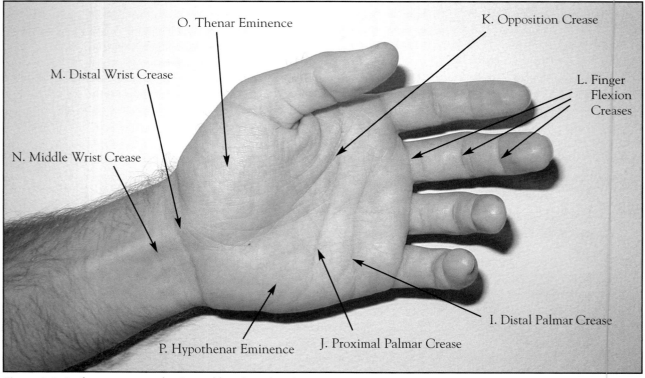

Figure 2-2. Surface anatomy of wrist and hand—volar view.

POSITIONS OF THE THUMB

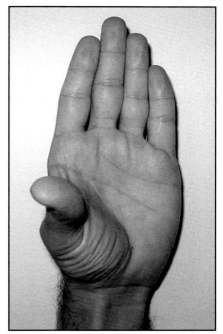

Figure 2-3. Abduction of the thumb.

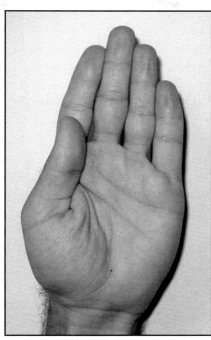

Figure 2-4. Adduction of the thumb.

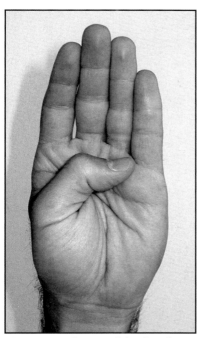

Figure 2-5. Flexion of the thumb.

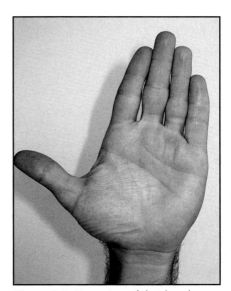

Figure 2-6. Extension of the thumb.

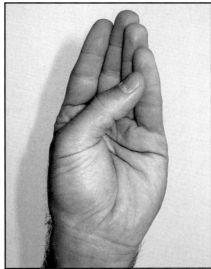

Figure 2-7. Opposition of the thumb.

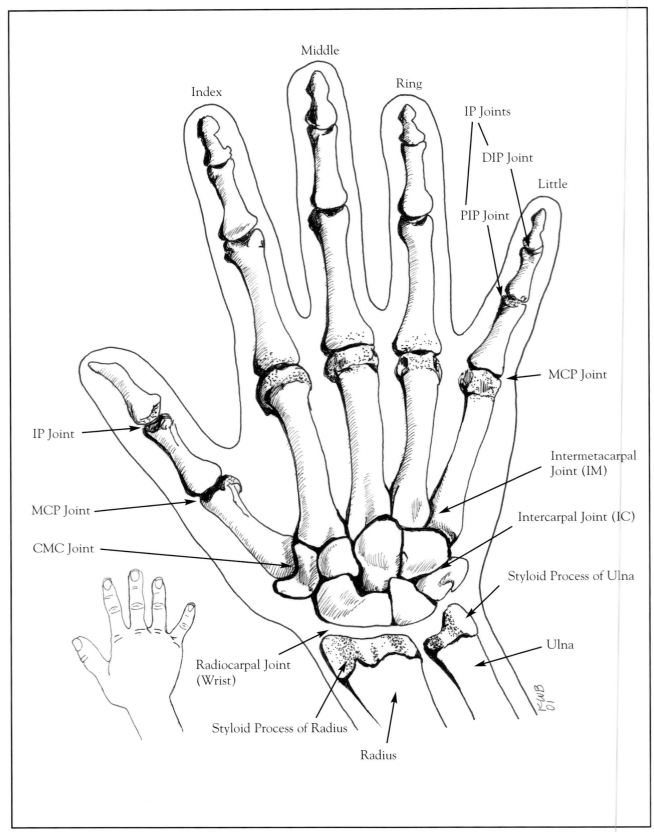

Figure 2-8. Bones of the right wrist and hand—dorsal view.

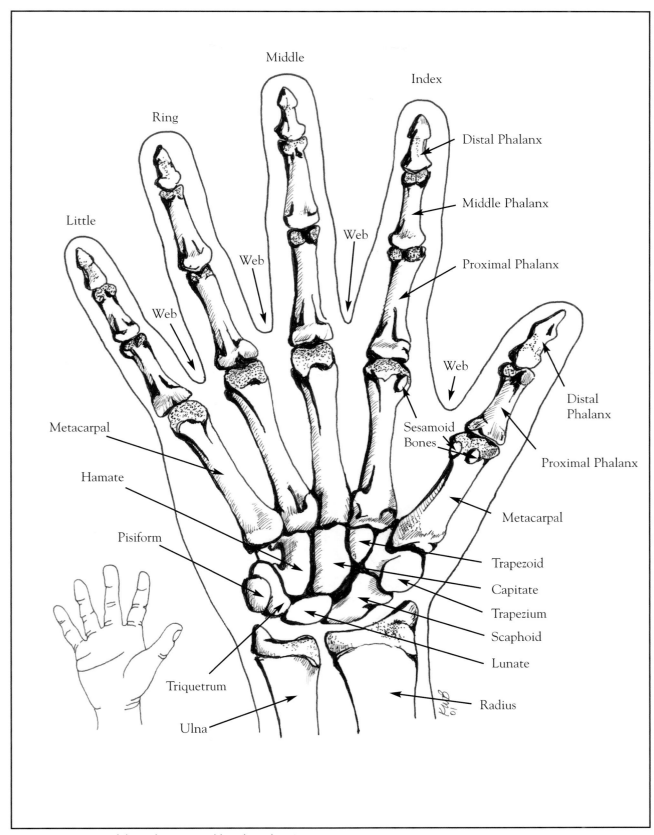

Figure 2-9. Bones of the right wrist and hand—volar view.

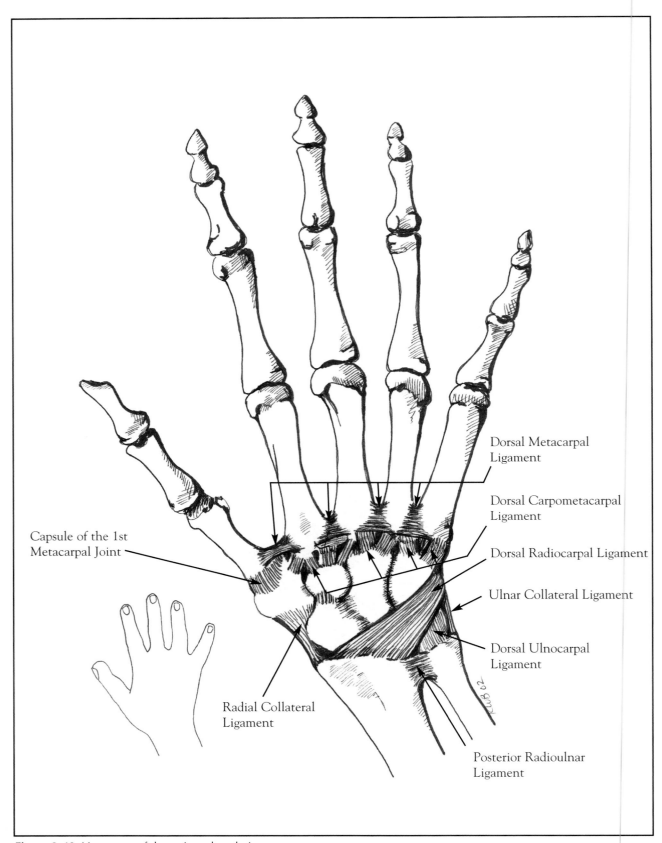

Figure 2-10. Ligaments of the wrist—dorsal view.

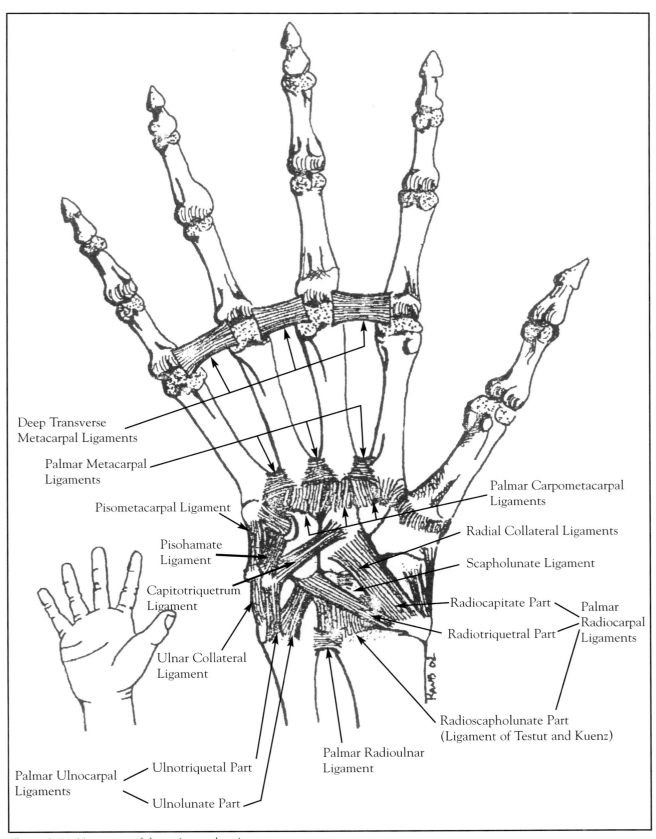

Deep Transverse
Metacarpal Ligaments

Palmar Metacarpal
Ligaments

Pisometacarpal Ligament

Pisohamate
Ligament

Capitotriquetrum
Ligament

Ulnar Collateral
Ligament

Palmar Carpometacarpal
Ligaments

Radial Collateral Ligaments

Scapholunate Ligament

Radiocapitate Part

Radiotriquetral Part

Palmar
Radiocarpal
Ligaments

Radioscapholunate Part
(Ligament of Testut and Kuenz)

Palmar Ulnocarpal
Ligaments

Ulnotriquetal Part

Ulnolunate Part

Palmar Radioulnar
Ligament

Figure 2-11. Ligaments of the wrist—volar view.

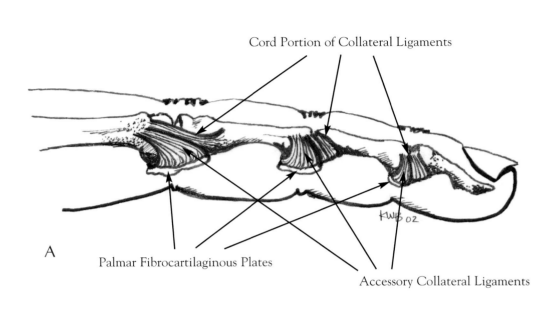

Cord Portion of Collateral Ligaments

Palmar Fibrocartilaginous Plates

Accessory Collateral Ligaments

A

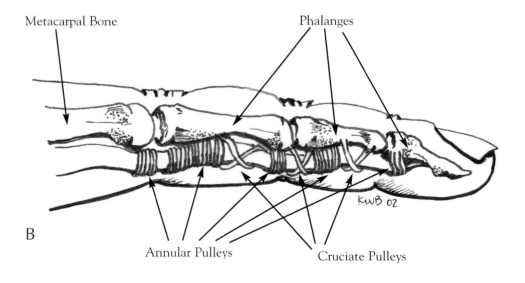

Metacarpal Bone

Phalanges

Annular Pulleys

Cruciate Pulleys

B

Figure 2-12. A: Ligaments of the digital joints. B: Digital flexor sheath.

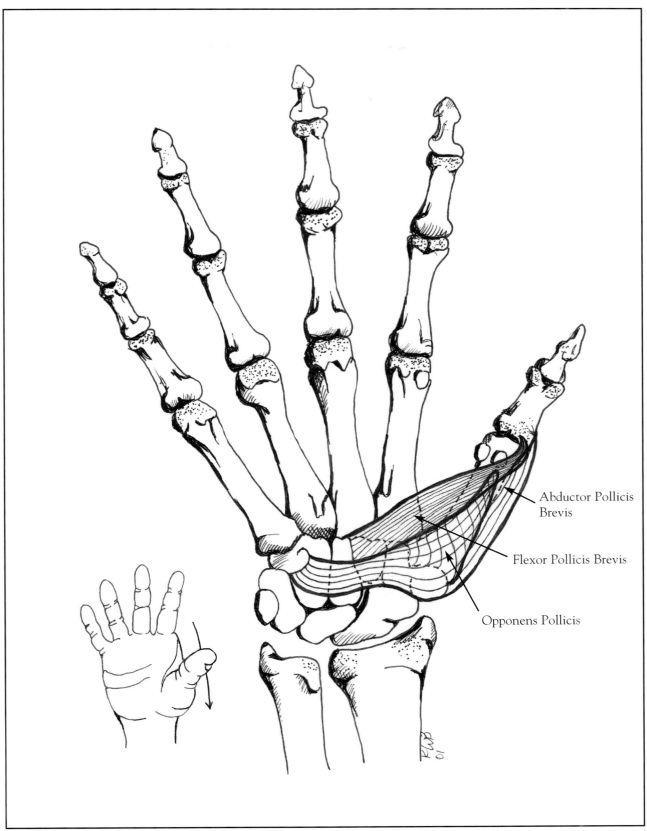

Figure 2-13. Intrinsic muscles of the thumb—abductor pollicis brevis, flexor pollicis brevis, and opponens pollicis.

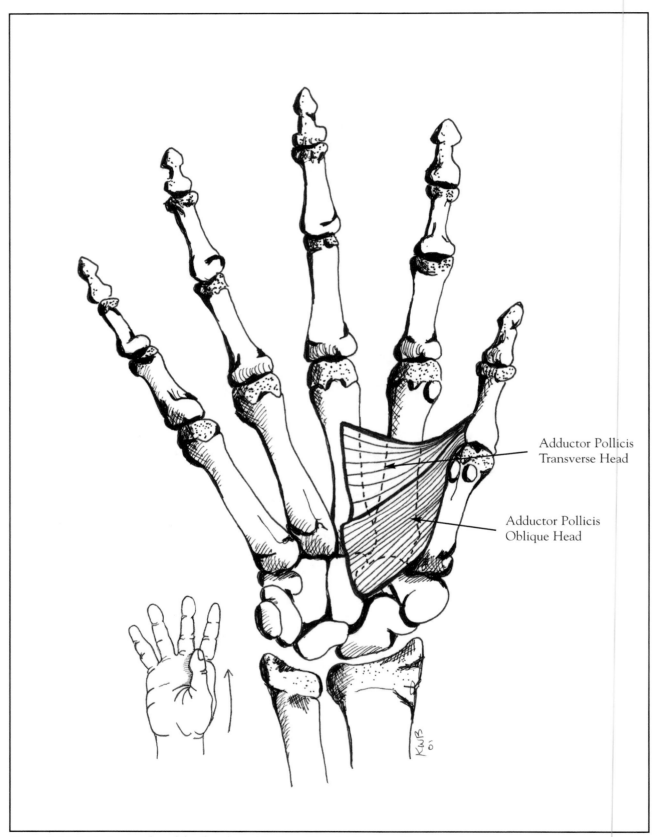

Adductor Pollicis
Transverse Head

Adductor Pollicis
Oblique Head

Figure 2-14. Intrinsic muscles of the thumb—adductor pollicis (oblique and transverse heads).

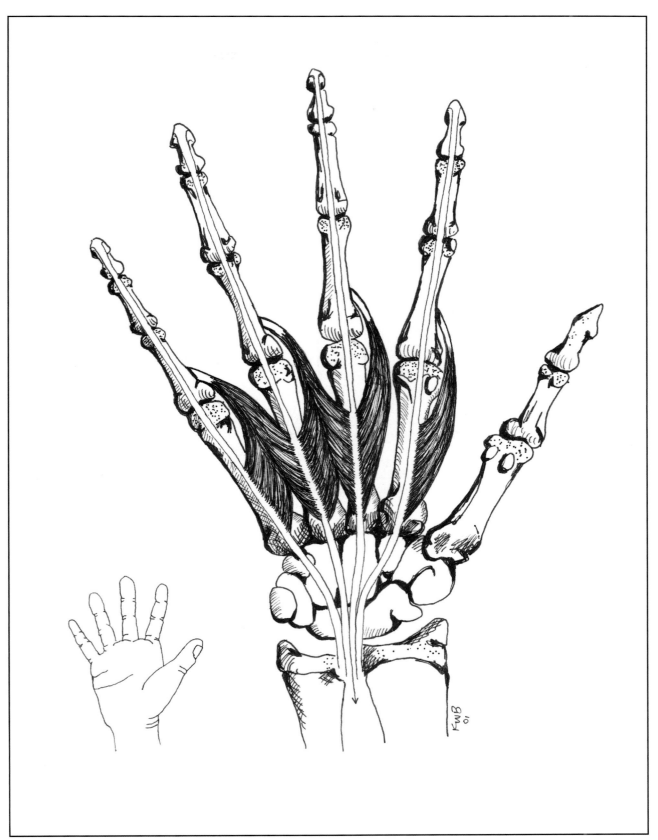

Figure 2-15. Intrinsic muscles of the palm of the hand—lumbricals.

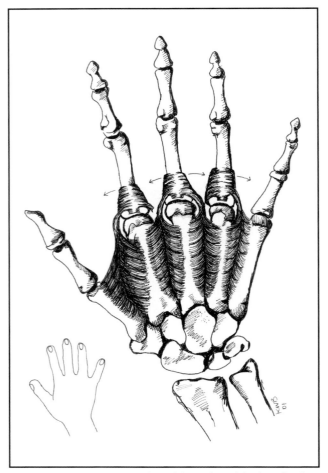

Figure 2-16. Intrinsic muscles of the palm of the hand—dorsal interossei.

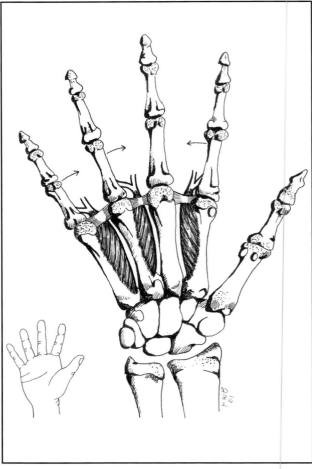

Figure 2-17. Intrinsic muscles of the palm of the hand—volar interossei.

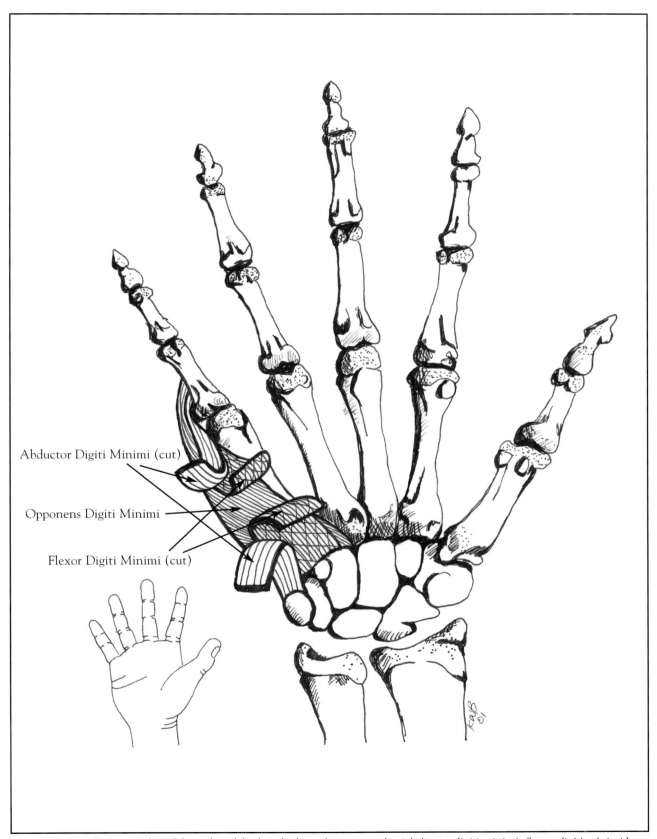

Figure 2-18. Intrinsic muscles of the palm of the hand—hypothenar muscles (abductor digiti minimi, flexor digiti minimi brevis, and opponens digiti minimi).

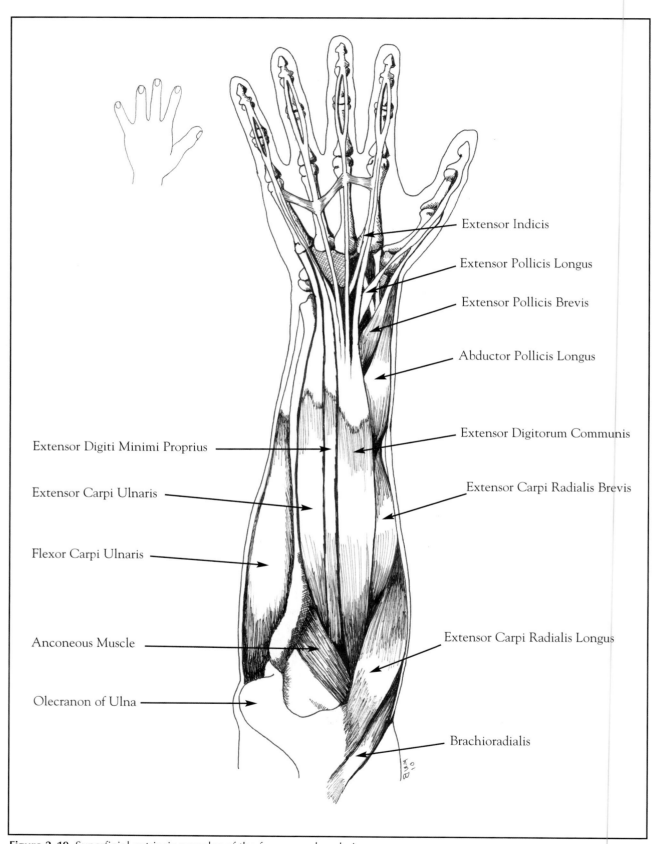

Extensor Indicis

Extensor Pollicis Longus

Extensor Pollicis Brevis

Abductor Pollicis Longus

Extensor Digitorum Communis

Extensor Digiti Minimi Proprius

Extensor Carpi Radialis Brevis

Extensor Carpi Ulnaris

Flexor Carpi Ulnaris

Anconeous Muscle

Extensor Carpi Radialis Longus

Olecranon of Ulna

Brachioradialis

Figure 2-19. Superficial extrinsic muscles of the forearm—dorsal view.

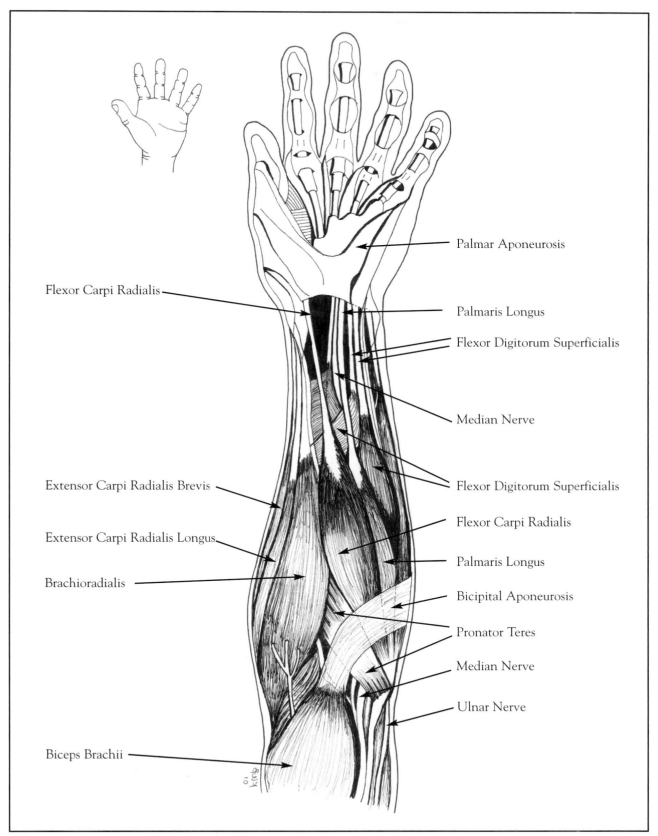

Figure 2-20. Superficial extrinsic muscles of the forearm—volar view.

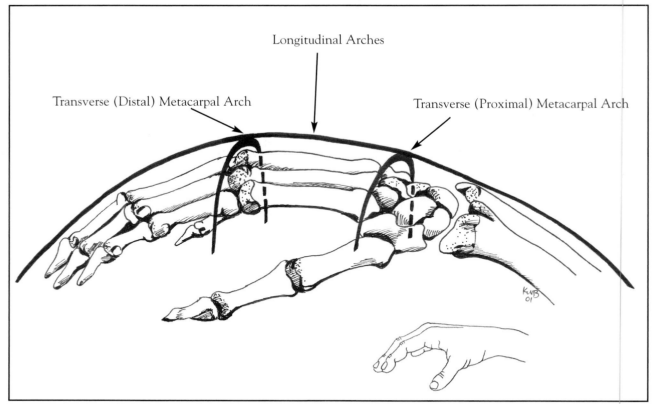

Figure 2-21. Longitudinal and transverse arches of the hand—lateral view.

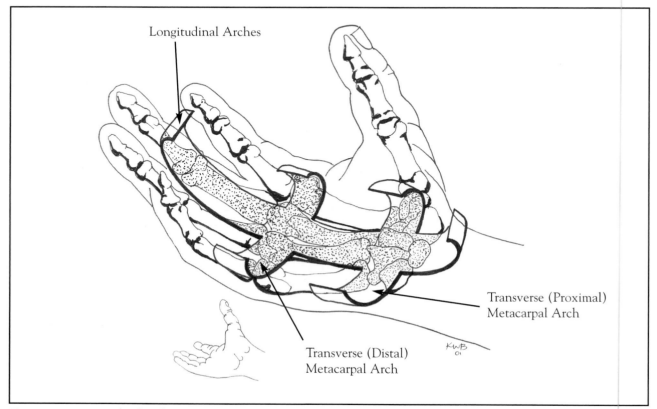

Figure 2-22. Longitudinal and transverse arches of the hand—palmar view.

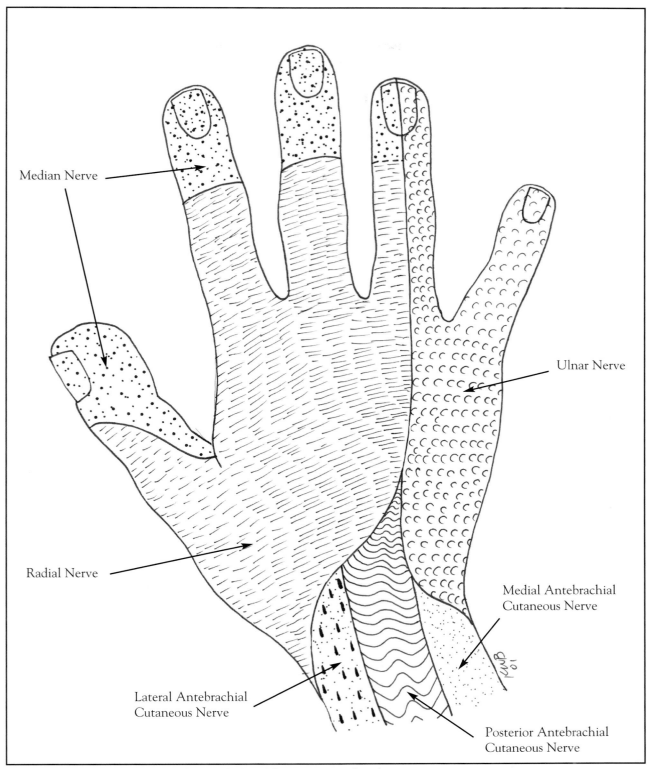

Figure 2-23. Innervation of the surface of the hand for sensation—dorsal view.

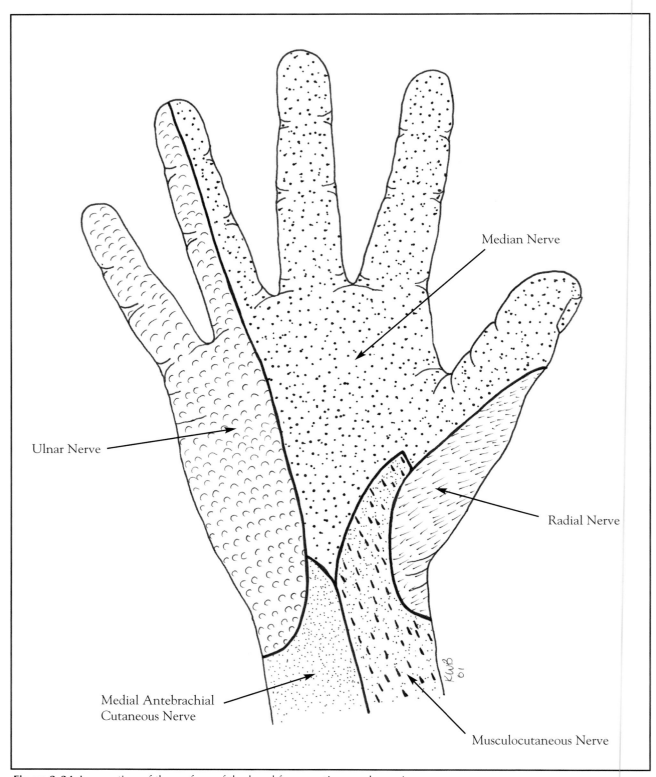

Figure 2-24. Innervation of the surface of the hand for sensation—palmar view.

CHAPTER THREE

REFLEXIVE BEHAVIORS THAT INFLUENCE GRASP

Reflexive behaviors are reactions that automatically occur as a response to sensory stimulation (Case-Smith, 1995). This sensory stimulation may be a particular head or body position (Fiorentino, 1981), as well as tactile input to an area of the skin. The result is a change in muscle tone that in turn affects posture and movement in consistent patterns. These patterns can be termed "reflexive behaviors," which may be defined as "a specific, automatic, patterned response that is elicited by a particular stimulus and does not involve any conscious control" (Fiorentino, 1981, p.13). Reflexes provide a range of movement experiences along with tactile and proprioceptive input (Case-Smith, 1995). Additionally, the reflexes that appear to have a connection with grasp emerge in a fairly orderly fashion in the typically developing infant, providing a means of assessment of the maturation of the infant and for the presence of acquired or congenital neurological delays (Twitchell, 1965b).

Research from the 1930s and 1940s has formed our understanding of reflex activity, but with current technology affording the opportunity to explore them in exciting news ways, our traditional understanding of reflexes has come into question. These early researchers concluded that young infants are capable of only reflexive movement (VanSant, 1994). Additionally, it was believed that early reflexes were "integrated, modified, and incorporated into more complex patterns in order to form the background for normal, voluntary movement and skills" (Fiorentino, 1981, p.ix). However, in recent years research has indicated that the fetus demonstrates the ability to move spontaneously throughout the fetal period before the reflexes emerge, questioning the validity of the assumption that the reflex is the basic unit of motor behavior and is a precursor of spontaneous movement (VanSant, 1994). Regardless of whether reflexes do or do not provide the background for volitional movement, it appears that early reflexes and purposeful grasp are clearly related.

The assumption of this relationship is based on clinical evidence that indicates if certain reflexes fail to develop, purposeful prehension will be adversely affected. Similarly, if certain reflexes emerge but become obligatory or do not integrate, prehension will be impaired (Twitchell, 1970). Ammon and Etzel (1977, p.13) indicate that "Even mild clumsiness in manipulation indicates a degree of disequilibrium in the development of the hand reflexes..." In addition, Twitchell (1970, p.34) states that "when none of the grasping automatisms develop, prehension is impossible." This illustrates the strength of the interrelationship between reflexes and prehension.

For these reasons, knowledge of expected reflex maturation is essential to understand the occurrence of deficits in reach and grasp (Ammon & Etzel, 1977). Reflexes need to be carefully evaluated in order to design successful intervention strategies when difficulty with the development of grasp is observed.

INTERRELATIONSHIP OF REFLEXES

The development of voluntary grasp is related to the automatic grasping reflexes (traction response, grasp reflex, and instinctive grasp reaction), and their equilibrium with the avoiding response (Twitchell, 1965b). The asymmetrical tonic neck reflex (ATNR) also plays a role in this process. The emergence and integration of these reflexes, along with the infant's interaction with the environment plays a vital role in the acquisition of hand skills.

An infant is typically born with the traction response (Twitchell, 1965b) and the ATNR (Simon & Daub, 1993). The avoiding response and the grasp reflex, both of which emerge during the first month of life, soon follow these early reflexes (Erhardt, 1994). Even for the newborn, these reflexes are helping provide movement experiences along with tactile and proprioceptive input (Case-Smith, 1995). For example, the presence of the ATNR encourages hand regard on the side of arm extension (Erhardt, 1994). When the infant begins to swipe at objects in the environment, it is with this extended arm that these movements occur. However, while the infant is beginning to demonstrate volitional movement towards a desired object, the infant's movements are still dominated by reflexive behaviors (in that as the arm extends, the traction response is elicited, causing the hand to become fisted as it approaches the desired object) (Ammon & Etzel, 1977).

By 3 to 4 months of age, the grasp reflex is fully developed and signals the emergence of more effective and persistent prehension (Twitchell, 1965b). At this time, the domination of the traction response is beginning to fade. As a result, the infant is beginning to isolate the grasping movements of the hand without the effect of the total flexion synergy of the traction response (Ammon & Etzel, 1977). However, even as the infant is gaining the ability to grasp with an open hand and extended elbow, the avoiding response interferes with these attempts at prehension. As the infant reaches for an object, the avoiding response causes extension and abduction of the fingers along with an overpronation of the hand. This results in a grasp on the ulnar side of the palm (Twitchell, 1970). This is considered a crude palmar grasp, and is typically seen during the 4th or 5th month of age (Gilfoyle, Grady, & Moore, 1990). The avoiding response also affects the grasp even after the object is secured, resulting in involuntary dropping of the object (Twitchell, 1970).

By 4 to 5 months of age, the grasp reflex has become altered so that when eliciting this reflex, slight orienting movements of the hand toward the contact stimulation are seen (Twitchell, 1965c). Twitchell (1965b) describes this as the orienting response, which is the earliest phase of the instinctive grasp reaction. The development of the instinctive grasp reaction enhances the infant's ability to orient the hand to an object in space, improving the effectiveness of reach and grasp (Twitchell, 1970). Because the instinctive grasp reaction enables the hand to adjust to the object being grasped, objects are (at this developmental level) grasped in the radial side of the hand using a superior [radial] palmar grasp (Ammon & Etzel, 1977). This grasp typically can be observed between the 6th and 7th month of age (Erhardt, 1994).

Between 8 and 10 months of age, the instinctive grasp reaction is fully developed (Duff, 1995). Fractionation of the grasp reflex, which typically begins to emerge at 4 months of age, is fully developed by 10 months of age. The maturation of these reflexes is necessary for the finger isolation and thumb opposition (Twitchell, 1965c) for precise prehension. Therefore, the full development of these reflexes precedes the emergence of the true [neat] pincer grasp (Twitchell, 1965c), which is typically seen between 10 and 12 months of age (Parks, 1988).

The following chapter is a description of five of the reflexes that influence volitional reach and grasp (Table 3-1). It is designed to describe these reflexive behaviors and to correlate that information to the infant's ultimate acquisition of prehension.

Table 3-1

REFLEX SUMMARY

Reflex	Initiation	Integration	Stimulus	Response
ATNR	Present at birth.	Between 4 and 6 months of age.	Head is turned to the right or left.	Limbs move into a flexion pattern on the side of the skull, or an extension pattern toward the side the face is turned.
Traction Response	Present at birth.	Between 2 and 5 months of age.	Passive stretch of the shoulder adductors and arm flexors, accomplished by pulling on the arm. Within a few weeks, a pressing stimulus to the palm elicits this reflex.	Flexion of the shoulder, elbow, wrist, and fingers.
Avoiding Response	Emerges during the 1st month of life.	At approximately 6 months of age, although remnants can be observed during life.	Light, distally moving contact to the hand.	Extension and abduction of fingers, withdrawal of hand from the stimulus.
Grasp Reflex	Emerges during the 1st month of life. Fractionation of this reflex begins to emerge at 4 months of age.	Between 6 and 9 months of age. Fractionation is fully developed by 10 months of age.	Deep pressing stimulus to the palm. The fractionated grasp reflex is elicited by a deep pressing stimulus to any one finger.	Sudden flexion/adduction of all of the joints of the fingers. Fractionated grasp reflex is seen as an isolated flexion of the stimulated finger.
Instinctive Grasp Response	Orienting stage emerges between 4 and 5 months of age.	By 10 months of age, the stimulus does not result in involuntary grasping. However, remnants can persist into adulthood.	Light contact stimulus to the radial or ulnar sides of the palm.	Supination or pronation (orienting) toward the stimulated side of the palm.
	Groping stage emerges between 6 and 7 months of age.			The orienting reaction followed by groping movements toward the stimulus.
	Trapping stage emerges between 8 and 10 months of age.			Orienting and groping reactions followed by grasping of the object.

Data from Twitchell, 1965a, 1965b, 1970; Ammon & Etzel, 1977; Simon & Daub, 1993; Erhardt, 1994; Duff, 1995; Murray, 1995.

PICTORIAL SUMMARY OF REFLEXES

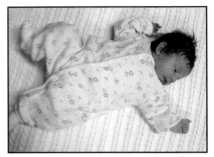

Asymmetric Tonic Neck
Reflex, pg. 35

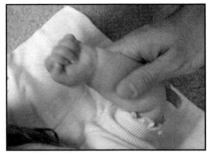

Traction Response, pg. 36

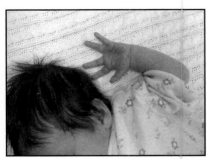

Avoiding Response, pg. 37

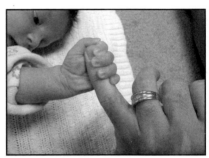

Grasp Reflex, pg. 38

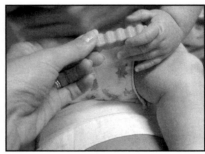

Instinctive Grasp Reaction,
pg. 39

ASYMMETRICAL TONIC NECK REFLEX (ATNR)

Initiation/Appearance

Present at birth (Simon & Daub, 1993). The peak incidence of this reflex is seen between 1 and 2 months of age (Barnes, Crutchfield, & Heriza, 1978).

Integration

Integrates between 4 and 6 months of age (Simon & Daub, 1993).

Central Nervous System Location

The ATNR is a brainstem reflex (Fiorentino, 1973).

Stimulus

Head is turned to the left or right (Murray, 1995).

Response

Limbs move into a flexion pattern on the skull side, and an extension pattern on the side toward which the face is turned (Fiorentino, 1973).

Significance to Grasp

The ATNR not only breaks the symmetrical flexion/extension pattern of movement, but it facilitates the separate use of each side of the body. This assists the infant with neck turning, visual fixation, and reaching. The aforementioned skills are building blocks to visually directed reaching and eye-hand coordination, both of which are essential components of grasping (Fiorentino, 1981).

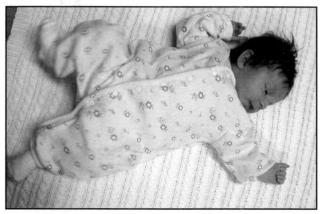

Figure 3-1. Note the extension of the upper and lower extremities on the side to which the face is turned, and the flexion of the upper and lower extremities on the opposite side of the body.

Interesting Information

The persistence of this reflex beyond an appropriate age or an obligatory response to the aforementioned stimulus affects functional grasp.

A persistent ATNR can compromise eye-hand coordination and midline orientation (Erhardt, 1994) and impact skills such as crossing the midline (Fiorentino, 1981), transferring objects, bringing toys or hands to the mouth (Gilfoyle et al., 1990), touching and exploring the body, and other manipulation skills. All of these skills are necessary building blocks for developing body image, self-feeding, and dressing (Barnes et al., 1978).

TRACTION RESPONSE

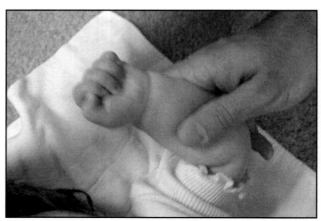

Figure 3-2. Note the flexion synergy of the traction response elicited by proprioception only (proprioceptive phase).

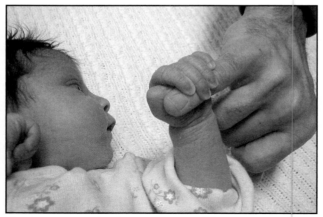

Figure 3-3. Note the flexion synergy of the traction response elicited by stimulation to the palm (contactual phase). This phase in the traction response also represents the earliest phase of the grasp reflex.

Initiation/Appearance

Proprioceptive Phase (Ammon & Etzel, 1977): Present at birth, and can be seen through 2 months of age (Twitchell, 1970).

Contactual Phase (Ammon & Etzel, 1977): Emerges between 2 and 4 weeks of age, and can be seen throughout the first few months of life (Twitchell, 1970).

Integration

Integrates between 2 and 5 months (Simon & Daub, 1993).

Central Nervous System Location

Originates in the pons (Simon & Daub, 1993).

Stimulus

Proprioceptive Phase: (Present at birth, and can be seen through 2 months of age.) The adequate stimulus to produce a response is passive stretching of the shoulder flexors and adductors accomplished by pulling on the arm (Twitchell, 1970).

Contactual Phase: (Emerges between 2 and 4 weeks of age, and can be seen throughout the first few months of life.) The traction response during this phase can be elicited by a deep pressing stimulus moving distally along the radial palm. Within a few weeks of the emergence of this phase, the traction response can also be elicited by contact stimulus drawn out between the thumb and index finger (Twitchell 1970).

Response

Proprioceptive Phase: (Present at birth, and can be seen through 2 months of age.) During this phase of the response, the stimulus results in the simultaneous flexion of the shoulder, elbow, wrist, and fingers (Ammon & Etzel, 1977).

Contactual Phase: (Emerges between 2 and 4 weeks of age, and can be seen throughout the first few months of life.) During this phase of the traction response, the stimulus drawn out between the thumb and index finger will produce an *immediate* flexion and adduction of the digits *followed by* flexion of the joints of the arm. The flexion of the joints of the arm is the traction response. The immediate flexion/ adduction of the digits constitutes the earliest phase in the emergence of the grasp reflex (Twitchell, 1970).

Significance to Grasp

An integrated traction response is necessary for an open hand during voluntary reach. Therefore, a persistence of this reflex will inhibit voluntary reach and grasp (Barnes et al., 1978). In addition, if the traction response is not integrated appropriately, an object placed in a child's hand will be pulled close to the child's body, inhibiting visual exploration and object manipulation (Gilfoyle et al., 1990).

Interesting Information

Between 2 and 2.5 months of age, an infant will fixate on a visual stimulus and swipe at or fling an arm toward the object. This swiping movement elicits the traction response by stretching the shoulder adductors, which causes the hand to become fisted (Ammon & Etzel, 1977).

At 3 months, the traction response has somewhat subsided, so the infant swipes with a hand that is more open. This is possible because the stretch to the shoulder flexors no longer produces a total flexion response. By 5 months, integration of the traction response allows the hand to be completely open during reaching (Ammon & Etzel, 1977).

AVOIDING RESPONSE

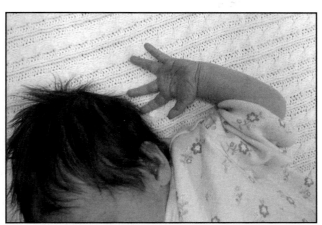

Figure 3-4. Note the extension and wide abduction of the fingers during the avoiding response.

Initiation/Appearance

Neonatal Phase: Appears between birth and 1 month of age (Erhardt, 1994).

Facile Phase: Emerges at approximately 1 to 2 months of age (Erhardt, 1994).

Integration

The avoiding response is integrated at approximately 6 months of age. At that time, the stimulus does not result in the withdrawal response. However, remnants of the avoiding response can be observed in children and adults under stress (Erhardt, 1994).

Central Nervous System Location

The origin of this reflex is subcortical (Simon & Daub, 1993).

Stimulus

Neonatal Phase: (Appears between birth and 1 month of age.) This response is difficult to elicit. The required stimulus is light contact moving distally along any part of the hand (Ammon & Etzel, 1977).

Facile Phase: (Emerges at approximately 1 to 2 months of age.) The response is easily elicited during this phase (Ammon & Etzel, 1977). The required stimulus is either light contact moving distally over the dorsal aspect of the hand and fingers, over the ulnar border of the hand, or to the pads of the fingertips (Ammon & Etzel, 1977).

Note: Both the neonatal phase and the facile phase of the avoiding response require a lighter contact stimulus than the grasp reflex (Twitchell, 1970).

Response

Neonatal Phase: (Appears between birth and 1 month of age.) This phase is characterized by a slight extension and abduction of the fingers (Ammon & Etzel, 1977).

Facile Phase: (Emerges at approximately 1 to 2 months of age.) This phase is characterized by finger extension and abduction, some wrist extension, forearm pronation, elbow flexion, and shoulder retraction (as if withdrawing the hand from a stimulus) (Ammon & Etzel, 1977).

Significance to Grasp

Finger flexion can be elicited with contact to the palm, allowing an object to be reflexively grasped when placed in the palm. However, the object will be dropped if it touches the fingertips, because that contact stimulus activates the avoiding response (Twitchell, 1970).

These avoiding responses cause ataxia of reach and overpronation of the hand during early attempts at voluntary prehension. As a result, objects are secured with the ulnar side of the hand, resulting in a [crude] palmar grasp (Twitchell, 1970).

The avoiding responses also help enable release of an object from the hand (Twitchell, 1970).

Interesting Information

The avoiding and grasping reactions emerge in an overlapping and orderly sequence (Twitchell, 1970).

As the initial component of the grasp reflex is appearing, an infant will alternately flex and extend the fingers—especially when excited. These movements are a result of the conflict between the grasp reflex and the avoiding response, which are not yet in equilibrium. These movements are commonly seen during the first year of life (Twitchell, 1970). Avoiding responses can affect posture and movement through early childhood. In fact, a remnant of the avoiding response can be seen as slight extension of the fingers following the appropriate stimulus and can persist throughout adulthood (Twitchell, 1970).

GRASP REFLEX

Initiation/Appearance

Grasp Reflex: Emerges during the natal period [first month of life] (Erhardt, 1994), and is fully developed by 3 to 4 months of age (Twitchell, 1965b).

Fractionated Grasp Reflex: Begins to emerge at 4 months, and is fully developed by 10 months of age (Twitchell, 1970).

Integration

The grasp reflex integrates between 6 and 9 months (Erhardt, 1994).

Central Nervous System Location

The sensory fibers arising from spinal cord levels C6 to C8 receive the sensory stimulus (Fiorentino, 1981) and the proprioceptive stimulus. The motor fibers that complete the reflex arc also arise from the same spinal cord levels (Fiorentino, 1981).

Stimulus

Grasp Reflex: (Emerges during the first month of life, and is fully developed by 3 to 4 months of age.) A deep pressing stimulus moving distally along the radial side of the palm elicits the fully developed grasp reflex (Twitchell, 1965b).

Fractionated Grasp Reflex: (Begins to emerge at 4 months, and is fully developed by 10 months of age.) When the grasp reflex is fully developed, it can be fractionated. In other words, a deep pressing stimulus to the volar aspect of any one of the fingers will elicit a response from only that finger (Ammon & Etzel, 1977).

Note: Deep pressing is important for both the grasp reflex and the fractionated grasp reflex, because if it is too light the stimulus will elicit an avoiding response (Twitchell, 1965b).

Response

Grasp Reflex: (Emerges during the first month of life, and is fully developed by 3 to 4 months of age.) A sudden flexion and adduction of all the joints of the fingers is seen, called the catching phase. This response can then be prolonged by traction on the fingers, called the holding phase (Twitchell, 1965a).

Fractionated Grasp Reflex: (Begins to emerge at 4 months, and is fully developed by 10 months of age.) A stimulus to any one of the fingers will elicit an isolated flexion of only that finger (Ammon & Etzel, 1977).

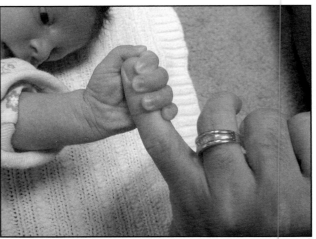

Figure 3-5. Note the flexion of the digits and the absence of the flexion synergy of the elbow and wrist in the grasp reflex. This contrasts with the traction response where the flexion pattern is observed not only in the digits, but also in the elbow and wrist.

Significance to Grasp

A persistent grasp reflex interferes with the ability to release objects (Gilfoyle et al., 1990). However, the presence of the avoiding reaction helps enable the release of objects from the hand. As these reactions emerge, an infant can be observed to flex and extend the fingers—especially when excited. These movements are the result of the interaction of the grasp reflex and avoiding response, which are not yet in equilibrium (Twitchell, 1970).

The fractionated grasp reflex helps enable flexion of one finger in isolation. This is an essential precursor to the ability to oppose any one finger to the thumb for fine manipulation. If this reflex fails to develop, manipulation of objects is clumsy (Twitchell, 1970).

Interesting Information

In its early phase, the grasp reflex is not entirely disassociated from the traction response. In fact, the stimulus to elicit the grasp reflex not only evokes the flexion/adduction of the fingers (which is the first phase in the development of the grasp reflex), but also elicits the flexion synergy of the upper extremity (which is a component of the traction response) (Twitchell, 1965b). However, when the grasp reflex is fully developed, the flexor synergy that characterizes the traction response can no longer be elicited (Twitchell, 1965c).

A purposeful grasp develops even before the grasp reflex is completely integrated (Fiorentino, 1981).

INSTINCTIVE GRASP REACTION

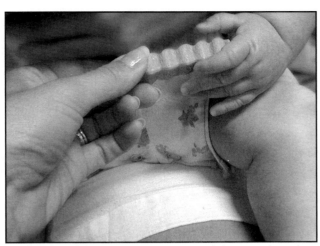

Figure 3-6. Note the supination toward the stimulus when the radial side of the hand is stimulated. This is the first phase in the instinctive grasp reaction.

Initiation/Appearance

Orienting Stage: Emerges between 4 to 5 months of age (Duff, 1995).

Groping Stage: Emerges between 6 to 7 months of age (Duff, 1995).

Trapping Stage: Emerges between 8 to 10 months of age (Duff, 1995).

Integration

By 10 months of age, the stimulus does not result in involuntary grasping (Erhardt, 1994). However, remnants of this reflex can persist into adulthood (Duff, 1995).

Central Nervous System Location

The origin of the instinctive grasp reaction is subcortical (Simon & Daub, 1993).

Stimulus

Orienting Stage: (Emerges between 4 and 5 months of age.) A light contact stimulus to the radial or ulnar sides of the hand elicits the orienting movements (Twitchell, 1965b).

Groping Stage: (Emerges between 6 and 7 months of age.) A light contact stimulus to the radial or ulnar sides of the hand elicits the groping movements (Twitchell, 1965b).

Trapping Stage: (Emerges between 8 and 10 months of age.) A light contact stimulus anywhere on the hand elicits the fully developed instinctive grasp reaction (Twitchell, 1965b).

Response

Orienting Stage: (Emerges between 4 and 5 months of age.) Supination toward the stimulated radial side of the hand or pronation toward the stimulated ulnar side of the hand (Twitchell, 1965b).

Groping Stage: (Emerges between 6 and 7 months of age.) The orienting reaction as described above followed by a movement toward the stimulus (Twitchell, 1965b).

Trapping Stage: (Emerges between 8 and 10 months of age.) The orienting and groping movements as described above followed by grasping of the object (Twitchell, 1965b).

Significance to Grasp

These responses assist the child in adjusting hand position according to the position of the object, improving efficiency and effectiveness of grasp patterns. The instinctive grasp reaction facilitates hand adjustments through tactile contact with an object, improving manipulative ability of the hands (Gilfoyle et al., 1990).

The early orientation phase of the instinctive grasp reaction enables the hand to readily adjust to the object, resulting in an attempt to grasp it with the radial side of the hand (Twitchell, 1970) using a superior [radial] palmar grasp (Ammon & Etzel, 1977).

Interesting Information

Without this reflex, more reliance is placed on visual guidance and cognitive attention to assist the child in orienting or adjusting his or her grasp to the shape of the object (Erhardt, 1994).

The instinctive grasp reaction is the most mature grasping reflex (Barnes et al., 1978).

Some fragments of the instinctive grasp reaction may persist into adulthood and are seen as a slight flexion of the fingers following an adequate contact stimulus (Twitchell, 1970).

CHAPTER FOUR

DEVELOPMENT OF GRASP

The transition from reflexive grasp patterns to purposeful grasp is an automatic, yet complicated process. It is difficult to determine when reflex activity no longer impacts grasp; there is not a clearly defined age or manner in which one can identify if reflexive behavior has been completely integrated. Pehoski (1992, p.1) states that the ability to use the hand "has a long developmental course," with the hands at birth being "crude instruments."

Motor control of the upper extremity is based on the principle of proximal and distal development. Kuypers states that "two distinct motor systems control the upper limbs; one proximal, is responsible for the control of large movements of arm and hand, the other distal, controls the subtle coordinations of hand movements" (Corbetta & Mounoud, 1990, p.191). It is thought that the proximal motor systems originate in brainstem structures, while the distal motor systems originate from cortical structures (Pehoski, 1992). Initially, a child's brainstem provides the proximal control of the upper limb to direct grasp. But as the child develops, control moves from the more basic centers of the brainstem to higher brain structures located in the cortex. The increasing role of the cortical structures provides the individualized finger control needed for precision grasping. This development progression of precise hand movements provides the neurological basis for the mass to specific pattern of development. The mass to specific pattern "indicates that less differentiated movement patterns precede discrete, highly specialized skills" (Exner,

2001, p.293). For example, the infant initially uses the whole hand (or palmar grasp) to pick up a block, which indicates that the infant has not gained the precise motor control necessary to use specialized hand skills, such as in a neat pincer grasp.

In addition to the neurological maturation that occurs as hand skills develop, many other factors must work together for optimal hand function. For example, postural control, motor planning, eye-hand coordination, tactile and proprioceptive input, and somatosensory processing also play a role in the development of a mature grasp. The maturation of grasp also depends on the underlying structures of the hand, such as the musculature, muscle tone, stability of the arches, and separation of the two sides of the hand. Therefore, when using this guide, one should be aware of the numerous factors that contribute to the developmental process.

The following chapter presents the typical developmental sequence of purposeful grasp (Table 4-1). The maturation of grasp should be considered a progression with overlapping sequences (Conner, Williamson, & Siepp, 1978). In other words, children do not typically master a new type of grasp and use it exclusively; experimentation and practice are common. Additionally, the ages presented here are approximate. Therefore, this progression should be used as a general guideline, taking into consideration the individuality of each child (Table 4-2).

COMPARISON OF DEVELOPMENTAL GRASP NAMES BY AUTHOR

Table 4-1

	Gilfoyle, Grady, & Moore, 1990	Johnson-Martin, Jens, Attermeier, & Hacker, 1991	Illingworth, 1991	Erhardt, 1994	Case-, Smith, 1995	Duff, 1995	Provence, Erikson, Vater, & Palmeri, 1995	Bruni, 1998	Case-Smith & Bigsby, 2000	Exner, 2001
Reflex Squeeze				Primitive squeeze	Primitive squeeze	Primitive squeeze				
Crude Palmar	Crude palmar		Palmar		Squeeze				Primitive squeeze	
Palmar				Palmar	Palmar	Palmar	Palmar	Palmar	Palmar	Palmar
Radial Palmar	Radial palmar			Radial palmar	Radial palmar	Radial palmar	Radial palmar		Radial palmar	
Raking Grasp				Inferior scissors						Crude raking
Radial Digital				Radial digital	Radial digital	Radial digital	Radial digital	Radial digital and Tripod	Radial digital	Radial digital
Developmental Scissors				Scissors	Scissors	Scissors	Scissors and Whole hand			
Inferior Pincer	Inferior pincer	Inferior pincer		Inferior pincer		Inferior pincer		Inferior pincer	Inferior pincer	
Three Jaw Chuck				3-Jawed chuck		Three jaw chuck				Three jaw chuck
Pincer			Superior pinch	Pincer		Pincer			Superior pincer	Pincer
Neat Pincer	Prehension	Neat pincer	Superior pincer	Fine pincer	Superior pincer	Superior pincer	Neat pincer	Superior pincer and Pinch		Tip pinch

Table 4-1

COMPARISON OF DEVELOPMENTAL GRASP NAMES BY AUTHOR, CONTINUED

	Halverson, 1931	Castner, 1932	Touwen, 1971	Gesell & Amatruda, 1974	Ammon & Etzel, 1977	Conner, Williamson, & Siepp, 1978	Newborg, Stock, Wnek, Guidubaldi, & Suinicki, 1984	Parks, 1988
Reflex Squeeze	Primitive squeeze				Primitive squeeze			
Crude Palmar	Squeeze	Whole-hand closure	Voluntary palmar		Squeeze			Ulnar palmar
Palmar	Palm and hand	Palmar prehension			Palmar			Palmar
Radial Palmar	Superior palm			Radial palmar	Superior palm			Radial palmar
Raking Grasp				Radial raking				Raking
Radial Digital	Inferior forefinger			Radial digital				Radial digital
Developmental Scissors		Scissors closure		Scissors	Inferior pincer			Prepincer and Inferior pinch
Inferior Pincer						Interior pincer		
Three Jaw Chuck	Forefinger				Forefinger			
Pincer		Pincer prehension		Inferior pincer				
Neat Pincer	Superior finger and Superior forefinger			Neat pincer	Neat pincer		Neat pincer	Neat pincer and Pincer

Table 4-2

COMPARISON OF DEVELOPMENTAL GRASP AGES BY AUTHOR

	Halverson, 1931	Castner, 1932	Gesell & Amatruda, 1974	Conner, Williamson, & Siepp, 1978	Parks, 1988	Gilfoyle, Grady, & Moore, 1990	Illingworth, 1991	Erhardt, 1994	Case-Smith, 1995	Duff, 1995	Provence, Erikson, Vater, & Palmeri, 1995	Exner, 2001
Reflex Squeeze	20 w (4 m)	20 w						4 m	20 w	20 w (5 m)		
Crude Palmar	20 to 24 w (4 to 5 m)	20 w.			3.5 to 4.5 m	Between 4 to 5 m			20 to 24 w			
Palmar	20 to 28 w (5 to 6 m)	32 to 36w	24 w		4 to 5 m			5 m	24 w	24 w (6 m)	4 to 7 m	By 6 m
Radial Palmar	24 to 32 w (6 to 7 m)	32 w	28 w		4.5 to 6 m			6 to 7 m	By 28 w	28 w (7 m)	4 to 7 m	
Raking Grasp	28 to 36 w (7 to 8 m)		32 w		7 to 8 m				7 m	7 m		7 m
Radial Digital	32 to 40 w (8 to 9 m)	36 w	36 w		7 to 9 m			8 m	9 m	36 w (9 m)	7 to 10 m	8 to 9 m
Developmental Scissors	32 to 40 w (8 to 9 m)	36 to 44 w	36 w		7.5 to 10 m			8 m	36 w	32 w (8 m)		
Inferior Pincer	32 to 40 w (8 to 9 m)			8 to 12 m		8 to 9 m		9 m	9 m	36 to 52 w, 9 to 12 m	7 to 10 m	
Three Jaw Chuck	44 to 52 w (10 to 12 m)	52 w						10 m		52 to 56 w, 1 year		
Pad to Pad	44 to 52 w (10 to 12 m)	52 w	40 w			10 to 12 m		10 m		38 to 52 w, 10 to 12 m		
Neat Pincer	44 to 52 w (10 to 12 m)	52w	48 w		10 to 12 m		9 to 10 m	12 m	12 m	52 to 56 w, 1 year	10 to 13 m	

w=weeks; m=months

PICTORIAL SUMMARY OF DEVELOPMENTAL GRASPS

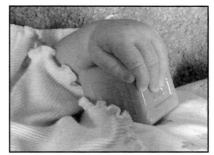

Reflex Squeeze Grasp, pg. 46

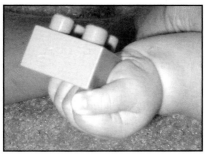

Crude Palmar Grasp, pg. 47

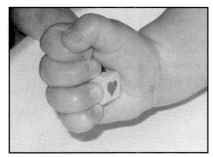

Palmar Grasp, pg. 48

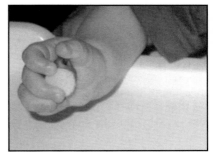

Radial Palmar Grasp, pg. 49

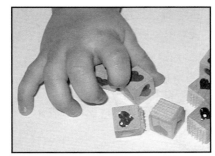

Raking Grasp, pg. 50

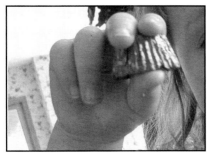

Radial Digital Grasp, pg. 51

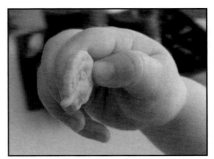

Developmental Scissors
Grasp, pg. 52

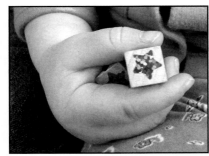

Inferior Pincer Grasp, pg. 53

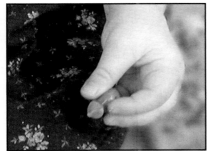

Three Jaw Chuck, pg. 54

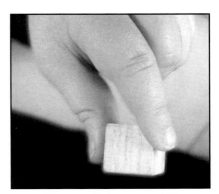

Pincer Grasp, pg. 55

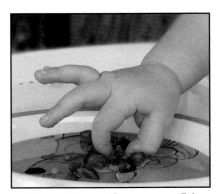

Neat Pincer Grasp, pg. 56

REFLEX SQUEEZE GRASP

Alternative Grasp Name

- *Primitive Squeeze Grasp* (Halverson, 1931; Ammon & Etzel, 1977; Erhardt, 1994; Case-Smith, 1995; Duff, 1995)

Description

Following the emergence of the grasp reflex, the infant begins to extend an arm toward a desired object but does not yet have the ability to purposefully grasp it in the hand. The infant's hand extends beyond the desired object (Halverson, 1931) and upon contact pulls the object back toward the body (Gilfoyle et al., 1990). The object is actually held between the hand and the body; this is not considered a true grasp as the hand is not actually grasping the object, but rather it is trapping it (Halverson, 1931). There is no thumb involvement with this grasp (Erhardt, 1994). Grasp at this age continues to be reflexive, and would be initiated by touching or moving an object through the hand (Case-Smith, 1995).

Age

This grasp is typically seen around 20 weeks or the 4th month of age.

Developmental Advancement

This pattern of corralling the object is adapted from swiping. Swiping, which represents a pattern of early reaching, can be seen between 2 and 2.5 months of age (Ammon & Etzel, 1977), when an infant will glance from

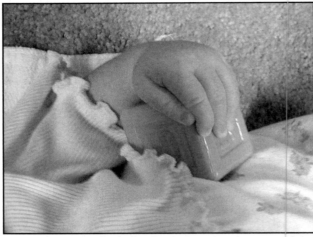

Figure 4-1. Note the lack of voluntary involvement of the thumb and the trapping of the object against the body, as opposed to actual prehension in the reflex squeeze grasp. Also, note the flexion of the wrist as the infant attempts to secure the object. This is a remnant of the traction response.

object to hand and attempt to contact the object with a full arm movement and closed fist (Gilfoyle et al., 1990). This closed fist is a result of the traction response, which is elicited during the extension of the arm during reach. As the child develops, the hand will be increasingly open during reach (Ammon & Etzel, 1977), helping to enable a true grasp. However, at this developmental stage a coordinated grasp has not developed.

CRUDE PALMAR GRASP

(Gilfoyle et al., 1990)

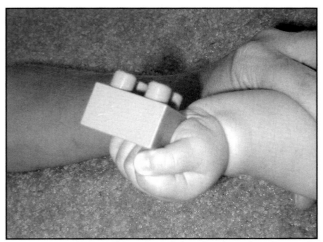

Figure 4-2. Observe the grasp of the object in the ulnar side of the palm and the lack of thumb involvement in this grasp.

Alternative Grasp Names

- *Squeeze Grasp* (Halverson, 1931; Ammon & Etzel, 1977; Case-Smith, 1995)
- *Whole-hand Closure* (Castner, 1932)
- *Voluntary Palmar Grasp* (Touwen, 1971)
- *Ulnar Palmar Grasp* (Parks, 1988)
- *Palmar Grasp* (Illingworth, 1991)
- *Primitive Squeeze* (Case-Smith & Bigsby, 2000)

Description

The crude palmar grasp typically follows the reflex squeeze grasp. The infant reaches out with a pronated forearm where, upon contact, simultaneous flexion of the fingers press the object firmly against the heel of the hand. The thumb is extended (Halverson, 1931) and does not play a role in pressing the object into the palm (Case-Smith, 1995). The infant's forearm is resting on a supported surface while actually grasping the object, but once the object is grasped the infant is able to pick up the object and bring it to midline for exploration. The infant is unable to open the hand in relation to the size or shape of the object as the fingers can only partially extend during the reaching pattern. As a result, the hand is placed crudely on the object (Gilfoyle et al., 1990). Finger differentiation is not present. Due to immature motor control and proprioceptive systems, the object is held tightly, which does not allow the object to move within the hand.

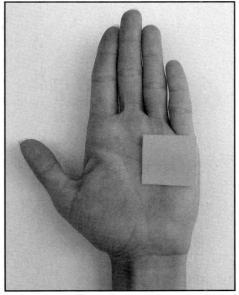

Figure 4-3. Illustration of object placement while using a crude palmar grasp (in the ulnar side of the palm).

This grasp is clumsy and is often unsuccessful (Case-Smith & Bigsby, 2000).

Age

This grasp is typically seen between 20 and 24 weeks or the 4th and 5th months of age.

Developmental Advancement

Reflexive patterns are becoming integrated and conscious grasp is beginning to take place (Ayres, 1954). The hand has developed the ability to grasp an object, although crudely. To facilitate the development of this grasp, an infant has built on the reflex squeeze grasp and scratching. Scratching is the alternating flexion and extension pattern of the fingers when in contact with various surfaces. Typically developed by 4 months, scratching helps an infant develop full range of reciprocal and combined finger flexion and extension, and provides tactile input to the fingers and palms of the hands (Gilfoyle et al., 1990). This tactile input and reciprocal movement patterns help promote greater awareness of the hand and contribute to the emergence of purposeful grasp.

PALMAR GRASP

(Ammon & Etzel, 1977; Parks, 1988; Erhardt, 1994; Case-Smith, 1995; Duff, 1995; Provence, Erikson, Vater, & Palmeri, 1995; Bruni, 1998; Case-Smith & Bigsby, 2000; Exner, 2001)

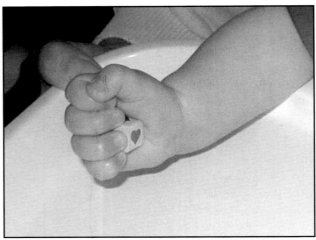

Figure 4-4. The object is secured in the center of the palm in the palmar grasp. Note the lack of participation of the thumb. Although the object is quite small, this infant has grasped it with the whole hand because he or she does not yet have the ability to prehend the object with more precise movements.

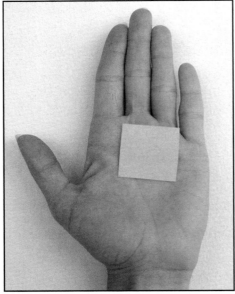

Figure 4-5. Illustration of object placement while using a palmar grasp (in the center of the palm).

Alternative Grasp Names

- *Palm Grasp* (Halverson, 1931)
- *Hand Grasp* (Halverson, 1931)
- *Palmar Prehension* (Castner, 1932)

Description

This grasp is characterized by the child putting the pronated hand down on the object, where the fingers flex simultaneously around the object to secure it in the midsection of the palm. The thumb is adducted and not assisting with the grasp (Erhardt, 1994; Case-Smith, 1995; Case-Smith & Bigsby, 2000). As the grasp matures, the object will move from the ulnar side of the hand toward the thenar eminence, and finally to the lower part of the thumb (Illingworth, 1963). In the early stages of this grasp, the forearm is in a pronated position (Case-Smith, 1995), which makes it difficult for the child to visualize the object so the child must rely on tactile cues for feedback about its position within the hand. "Grasp remains palmar regardless of size of object, so that even small objects are taken between fingers and palm and sometimes lost in the palm" (Gilfoyle et al., 1990, p. 163).

Age

This grasp is typically seen between 20 and 28 weeks or the 5th and 6th months of age.

Developmental Advancement

The forearm continues to be pronated impeding visual guidance. The forearm is positioned in pronation during the child's first reaching pattern, but by the 6th month, supination of the forearm increases, allowing the child to visualize the grasped object (Case-Smith, 1995). While using the palmar grasp, the infant grasps an object in the midsection of the palm. As maturation and greater motor control are gained, the radial side of the hand becomes more dominant, improving the success of the grasp. The shift to the radial side of the hand "foretells thumb opposition" (Gesell & Amatruda, 1974, p. 60).

RADIAL PALMAR GRASP

(Gesell & Amatruda, 1974; Parks, 1988; Gilfoyle et al., 1990; Erhardt, 1994; Case-Smith, 1995; Duff, 1995; Provence et al., 1995; Case-Smith & Bigsby, 2000)

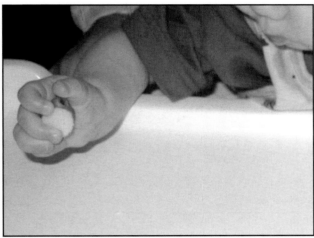

Figure 4-6. The object is secured in the radial side of the palm. Note the flexion of the ulnar fingers for stability and the thumb that is beginning to oppose and actively press the object into the palm.

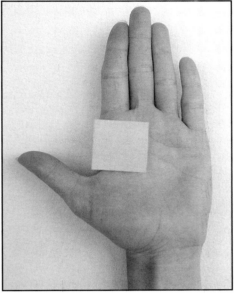

Figure 4-7. Illustration of object placement while using a radial palmar grasp (in the radial side of the palm).

Alternative Grasp Name

- *Superior Palm Grasp* (Halverson, 1931; Ammon & Etzel, 1977)

Description

In this grasp, the object is secured in the radial side of the palm. The index and middle fingers flex around the object, as the thumb begins to oppose the fingers to press the object into the radial palm.

As the grasp matures, the thumb becomes more active (Case-Smith, 1995). The two ulnar digits flex into the palm as they begin to act as a stabilizer for the now more dominant radial side. With the ulnar digits flexed into the palm to provide stability to the radial side of the hand, this grasp represents the earliest example of coupling (which is the differentiation in the function of the two sides of the hand). The object continues to be pressed into the palm, restricting the manipulative movements of higher-level grasps.

Age

This grasp is typically seen between 24 and 32 weeks or the 6th and 7th months of age.

Developmental Advancement

This grasp marks a significant change in the activity of the hand. The emergence of the instinctive grasp response allows the hand to adjust to the object being grasped. Therefore, objects are grasped in the radial side of the hand (Ammon & Etzel, 1977). This is also the beginning of thumb opposition, which is highly significant for the infant, as opposition is necessary for the continued development of the mature grasp and will be used throughout adulthood. Opposition, along with the prominence of the index finger, is largely responsible for the higher level grasps (Halverson, 1931). Another significant advancement is that the hand now has two definite sides, one that manipulates or grasps and one that stabilizes the movement. This grasp signifies the initial development of the radial side of the hand as the skill side of the hand (Case-Smith, 1995). This differentiation will eventually allow an infant to pick up and grasp two small objects simultaneously (Conner et al., 1978).

RAKING GRASP

(Parks, 1988)

Alternative Grasp Names
- *Radial Raking* (Gesell & Amatruda, 1974)
- *Inferior Scissors Grasp* (Erhardt, 1994)
- *Crude Raking* (Exner, 2001)

Description
The grasp is characterized by the child reaching for and grasping a small object using a raking motion (Erhardt, 1994). The hand is positioned in a rake-like manner with all of the fingers flexed at the IP joints. The fingers, hand, and arm move as one unit to "rake" the small object into the palm (Bruni, 1998). The hand may need support from a solid surface to be successful. This grasp is not always successful, and if it is, manipulation does not occur.

Age
This grasp is typically seen between 28 and 36 weeks or the 7th and 8th months of age.

Developmental Advancement
This raking motion provides important tactile contact with objects that helps stimulate sensory development, which is needed for the development of grasp.

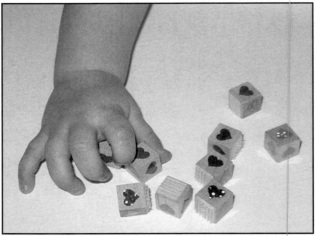

Figure 4-8. Note the flexion of the radial fingers to bring the objects into the palm while using the raking grasp.

RADIAL DIGITAL GRASP

(Gesell & Amatruda, 1974; Parks, 1988; Erhardt, 1994; Case-Smith, 1995;
Duff, 1995; Provence et al., 1995; Bruni, 1998; Case-Smith & Bigsby, 2000; Exner, 2001).

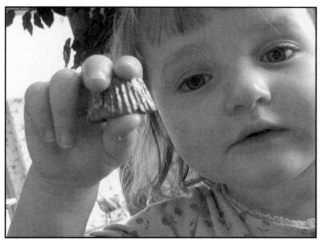

Figure 4-9. Observe the full opposition of the thumb to help secure the object, and the flexion of the ulnar fingers for stability while using the radial digital grasp.

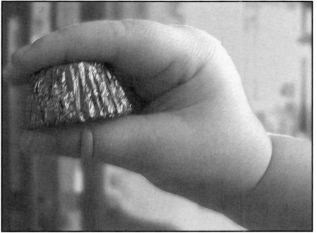

Figure 4-10. Note the space between the object and the palm in the radial digital grasp. Also note that the object is secured proximal to the fingertips because the fine motor control needed for a fingertip grasp has not yet developed. This grasp is differentiated from the three jaw chuck, in that the three jaw chuck uses the pads of the fingers and thumb to secure the object.

Alternative Grasp Names

* *Inferior Forefinger Grasp* (Halverson, 1931)
* *Tripod Grasp* (Bruni, 1998)

Description

This grasp is characterized by thumb opposition to the radial fingers. The object is held proximal to the pads of the fingers with space visible between the object and the palm. The ring and little finger are flexed. The forearm is in a neutral position when reaching, which provides greater visual direction for grasping. This grasp is similar to the radial palmar grasp, but now the object is held away from the palm, giving the child greater manipulative control. Yet, this grasp is not a fingertip grasp, because the object is held proximal to the pads of the fingers (Halverson, 1931). "[T]he infant can adjust the object within the hand and as a result can use the object for various purposes while holding it" (Case-Smith, 1995, p.117).

Age

This grasp is typically seen between 32 and 40 weeks or the 8th and 9th months of age.

Developmental Advancement

The fingers are beginning to gain the motor control and proprioceptive feedback needed to begin digital grasping. Sensory feedback is providing the hand with more discrete information, offering the hand increased control and precision. The fingers now have the ability to "maintain the delicately balanced pressure of the digits" (Halverson, 1931, p.218) necessary to secure an object. The developing motor control and proprioceptive systems provide a balance that gives the radial side of the hand the ability to begin to act independently of the palm and the ulnar fingers, giving the child the ability to grasp two objects in one hand (Case-Smith, 1995).

DEVELOPMENTAL SCISSORS GRASP

Alternative Grasp Names

- *Scissors Closure* (Castner, 1932)
- *Scissors Grasp* (Gesell & Amatruda, 1974; Erhardt, 1994; Case-Smith, 1995; Duff, 1995; Provence et al., 1995)
- *Inferior Pincer Grasp* (Ammon & Etzel, 1977)
- *Pre-Pincer Grasp* (Parks, 1988)
- *Inferior Pinch* (Parks, 1988)
- *Whole Hand Grasp* (Provence et al., 1995)

Description

This grasp is characterized by the object being secured between the adducted thumb and radial side of the flexed index finger. The thumb is not opposed, but slides over in a pattern of adduction to trap an object against the side of the index finger. "The thumb envelops rather than manipulates" (Ayres, 1954, p. 97). The ulnar digits are loosely flexed and do not flex or extend with the radial digits (Gesell & Amatruda, 1974); in the flexed position the ulnar digits provide stability for the radial side of the hand. The hand requires stabilization from a solid surface for successful grasping of the object. Castner (1932) named this grasp the scissors closure due to the similar action of the thumb being drawn to the index finger, mimicking the action of operating a pair of scissors.

Age

This grasp is typically seen between 32 and 40 weeks or the 8th and 9th months of age.

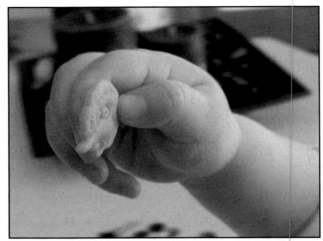

Figure 4-11. Note the adduction of the thumb to secure the object against the radial side of the index finger while using the developmental scissors grasp.

Developmental Advancements

The thumb is taking on a more independent role in the grasping process, as observed in the separate actions of the thumb and radial fingers. This independent action is necessary for more mature grasps. However, the thumb lacks the ability to oppose the digits, which is necessary for many precision grasps.

INFERIOR PINCER GRASP

(Conner et al., 1978; Gilfoyle et al., 1990; Johnson-Martin, Jens, Attermeier, & Hacker, 1991; Erhardt, 1994; Duff, 1995; Bruni, 1998; Case-Smith & Bigsby, 2000)

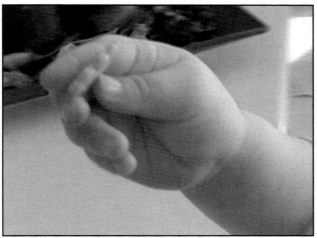

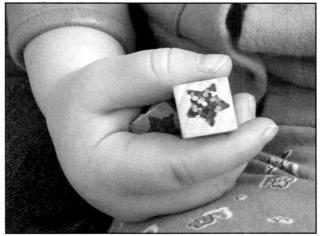

Figure 4-12. Note the adduction of the thumb to secure the object against the extended index finger while using the inferior pincer grasp.

Figure 4-13. This is an example of the inferior pincer grasp where the thumb has achieved full opposition (rotation and abduction of the thumb). However, the object is still held proximal to the fingertip. This grasp is differentiated from the radial digital grasp in that only two digits, the thumb and the index finger, are needed to secure the object.

Description

This grasp is characterized by thumb adduction and emerging opposition to secure the object against the extended index finger. The object is held proximal to the pad of the finger (Case-Smith, 1995). The extension of the index finger IP joints supports prehension, but not manipulation of the object (Gilfoyle et al., 1990). Depending on the degree of thumb opposition, MCP and IP flexion of the joint of the thumb will vary. The ulnar three digits are flexed toward the palm providing stability. The hand and arm continue to require support from the table to accomplish a successful grasp. At this age, the precision needed for a fingertip grasp has not been developed.

Age

This grasp is typically seen between 32 and 40 weeks or the 8th and 9th months of age.

Developmental Advancements

The grasp is usually adapted from index finger probing (Case-Smith, 1995), a nonprehensile movement pattern that isolates extension of the index finger with the ulnar digits flexed for stability (Gilfoyle et al., 1990). This beginning of index finger isolation, together with a thumb to finger pattern of movement, is fundamental to more mature patterns of prehension (Gilfoyle et al., 1990).

This grasp should not be underestimated in terms of its significance to the development of prehension because the inferior pincer grasp represents the beginning stage of opposition. The continued development of opposition helps enable the child to prehend small objects with increasingly greater precision and control.

THREE JAW CHUCK

(Duff, 1995; Exner, 2001)

Alternative Grasp Names

- *3-Jawed Chuck Grasp* (Erhardt, 1994)
- *Forefinger Grasp* (Halverson, 1931; Ammon & Etzel, 1977)

Description

This grasp is characterized by thumb opposition to the index and middle fingers. The object is held at the pads of the index and middle fingers, as well as the pad of the thumb. The IP joints of the index and middle fingers range from extended to slightly flexed, with flexion of the MCP joints. To oppose the digits, the thumb rotates and flexes toward the fingertips. The ulnar two digits do not participate in grasping the cube, but provide support to the radial side of the hand. A solid surface serves as a "leverage point for lifting the hand after it grasps the cube" (Halverson, 1931, p. 219).

Age

This grasp is typically seen between 44 and 52 weeks or the 10th and 12th months of age.

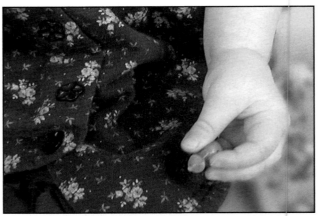

Figure 4-14. Note the full opposition of the pad of the thumb to the pad of both the index and middle fingers while using the three jaw chuck.

Developmental Advancements

This grasp marks the beginning of the tripod posture, which is used for writing and many other tasks. The radial digits no longer flex around the object (Halverson, 1931); instead the pads of the fingers and thumb secure the object. Proprioceptive feedback from these digits enables the fingers and thumb to provide the appropriate pressure needed to secure the object.

PINCER GRASP

(Erhardt, 1994; Duff, 1995; Exner, 2001)

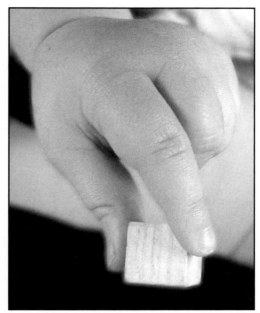

Figure 4-15. Note the full opposition of the pad of the thumb and the pad of the index finger to secure the object while using the pincer grasp. This is differentiated from the neat pincer grasp, in that the pad of the finger secures the object in the pincer grasp; whereas the tip of the finger secures the object in the neat pincer grasp.

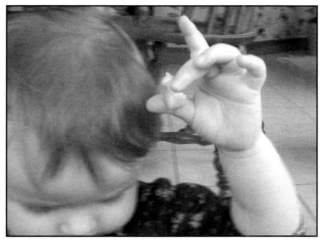

Figure 4-16. This is an example of the pincer grasp in which the pad of the middle finger is securing the object against the thumb.

Alternative Grasp Names

- *Pincer Prehension* (Castner, 1932)
- *Inferior Pincer Grasp* (Gesell & Amatruda, 1974)
- *Superior Pinch* (Gilfoyle et al., 1990)
- *Superior Pincer Grasp* (Case-Smith & Bigsby, 2000)

Description

This grasp is characterized by the object being held between the opposed thumb and pad of the index or middle finger. The MCP and IP joints of the thumb are extended. The index finger is flexed at the MCP, slightly flexed at the PIP and extended at the DIP. The finger and thumb usually come together in the vertical plane (Castner, 1932) with the forearm in the midposition, offering the child increased visual regard. When grasping the object, the child rests only the fingertips on the tabletop for support.

Age

This grasp is typically seen between 44 and 52 weeks or the 10th and 12th months of age.

Developmental Advancements

Minimal external support is needed with the grasp. Hirschel, Pehoski, and Coryell (1990) state that with increased age children develop internal stability, which enables them to grasp with progressively less external support. The developmental progression of forearm position allows the child greater visual regard of the object, which assists in precision grasping.

NEAT PINCER GRASP

(Gesell & Amatruda, 1974; Ammon & Etzel, 1977; Newborg, Stock, Wnek, Guidubaldi, & Suinicki, 1984; Parks, 1988; Johnson-Martin et al., 1991; Provence et al., 1995)

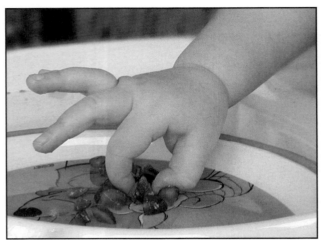

Figure 4-17. Note the flexion of all of the joints in the thumb and index finger so that the tip of the finger and the thumb come together to prehend very small objects. The neat pincer grasp is differentiated from the pincer grasp, in that the pincer grasp uses the pad of the index finger to secure the object as opposed to using the tip of the finger.

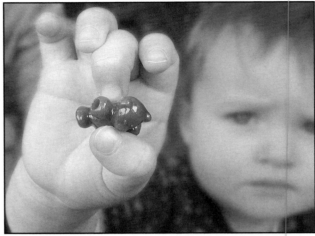

Figure 4-18. This is an example of the tip of the middle finger and the thumb securing a small object.

Alternative Grasp Names

- *Superior Forefinger Grasp* or *Superior Finger Grasp* (Halverson, 1931)
- *Pincer Grasp* (Parks, 1988)
- *Prehension* (Gilfoyle et al., 1990)
- *Superior Pincer Grasp* (Illingworth, 1991; Case-Smith, 1995; Duff, 1995; Bruni, 1998)
- *Fine Pincer Grasp* (Erhardt, 1994)
- *Tip Pinch* (Exner, 2001)
- *Pinch* (Bruni, 1998)

Description

This grasp is characterized by the object being held between the opposed thumb and the fingertip of the index or middle finger. All joints of the index or middle fingers are flexed. The longitudinal arch is aligning the phalanges and the MCP joint, which supports this position. The child no longer requires support from a solid surface. The forearm is in the midposition, enabling the child to visually guide the hand toward the object.

Age

This grasp is typically seen between 44 and 52 weeks or the 10th and 12th months of age.

Developmental Advancements

The child no longer needs external support to successfully grasp an object, indicating continued development of internal stability. Greater control of finger flexion and extension also allows the child to bring the fingertip to the thumb for precision grasping. This ability to fractionate the flexion and extension of the IP joints of the fingers is essential for manipulation.

CHAPTER FIVE

GRASPS FOR HANDWRITING

Handwriting is a lifetime activity and each person has a unique and individual style. The most common pencil grasps used for handwriting are presented in this chapter. These grasps are presented in three phases of developmental progression, moving from the primitive or immature grasp pattern to the transitional grasp phase to the mature grasp pattern. This progression is not linear; as children develop new skills they will use familiar grasp patterns and experiment with new ones. All of the grasps presented in this chapter can be observed in young children, but certainly not every child will use each grasp (Schneck & Henderson, 1990). The progression through these developmental stages is very individualized and therefore, this chapter is intended to be a general guideline.

Handwriting is a complex task that involves moving a pencil in specific directions to achieve a desired outcome. It is a dynamic task that requires more than an efficient pencil grip (Penso, 1990). Research of handwriting has documented that specific skills, such as in-hand manipulation, visual-motor skills, visual perception, fine motor, and perceptual motor skills are linked to successful handwriting (Case-Smith, 2002). It is important to include these components in an evaluation of handwriting. A thorough evaluation would also include additional sensorimotor functions, such as posture, bilateral integration, motor planning, kinesthesia, tactile and proprioceptive

feedback, and balance. The precise movements of the hand needed for handwriting also depend on the development of the musculature and supporting structures of the hand, stability of the arches and wrist, and separation of the two sides of the hand. Other factors, such as upper extremity strength and endurance are also important for the controlled movement needed for legible handwriting.

Another important factor in the acquisition of handwriting is the principle of proximal *and* distal development. This is important to pencil grasps because the initial stability needed for controlled arm mobility originates in the trunk and shoulder. Posture and the "integration of movements of the body and the limbs" are controlled by the brainstem, but fragmented finger movements are controlled by the motor cortex through the corticospinal tracts (Pehoski, 1992, p. 2). Because the corticospinal tracts are not completely myelinated until about age 3 (Pehoski, 1992), a child will initially rely on the larger muscle groups of the arm to control the pencil. A child, using a primitive grasp, will initially use the trunk and whole arm to move the pencil across the paper. As the central nervous system matures, the child begins to rely less on the trunk for stability and control of the pencil, and relies more on distal musculature and external support. This change in the locus of stability can be seen in transitional grasps when the elbow and wrist gain more control, while the forearm begins to rest on the tabletop (which acts as an external stabilizer). The hand soon gains the neural control needed for individual finger mobility, which provides greater control over the pencil. This combination of neurological and muscular maturation guides the proximal and distal progression of the pencil grasp pattern. With the above mechanisms in place, a mature grasp pattern will have a combination of a stable elbow and wrist in order to allow for shoulder mobility and discrete finger movements (Exner, 2001).

These components of handwriting are developed by neurological maturation and years of practice. However, this developmental process can be influenced by various environmental factors, such as the opportunity to use writing utensils, the value caregivers place upon acquisition of handwriting skills, as well as gender and cultural influences. Research indicates that boys and girls differ in the pencil grasp patterns used (Schneck and Henderson, 1990; Summers, 1990). Saida and Miyashita (1979) found that girls develop a dynamic tripod approximately 6 months earlier than boys and that Japanese children adopt the dynamic tripod earlier than their European and American counterparts. The latter is possibly the result of Japanese children's use of chopsticks and the consequential "opportunity to manipulate objects in an advanced manner of prehension" (Saida & Miyashita, 1979, p. 112). This experience may help enable them to gain the fine motor skills required to use the dynamic tripod earlier than children of other cultures.

Although the dynamic tripod grasp is thought to be the most efficient, skilled, and desirable grasp pattern, research has not shown that the use of this grasp improves handwriting performance (Schneck, 1991). Ziviani and Elkins (1986) state, "there is a degree of individual variation which is apparently not detrimental to the performance of a task [of handwriting]" (p. 256). When comparing the dynamic tripod grasp with transitional grasps or other mature grasp patterns, it has been found that speed (Sassoon, Nimmo-Smith, & Wing, 1986; Ziviani & Elkins, 1986); and legibility are not affected by grasp (Ziviani & Elkins, 1986; Dennis & Swinth, 2001). Additionally, Bergmann (1990) suggests that mature movement patterns are more important than a particular grasp pattern, implying that a specific grasp is unlikely the sole cause of poor handwriting. Therefore, when evaluating handwriting, it is important to have an understanding of the developmental progression of grasp as well as the muscular and movement patterns involved with each pencil grasp.

Pencil grasps are divided into groups that are considered to be primitive, transitional, or mature (Schneck &

Henderson, 1990). This chapter is organized according to these divisions.

Primitive grasps, or immature grasp patterns, hold the pencil in the palm in a power-type grasp. The forearm may or may not be resting on the table. The movement of the pencil is achieved by a combination of wrist, arm, and trunk movements; finger or thumb movements are not typically seen (Elliott & Connolly, 1984). Primitive grasps are typically seen before 4 years of age (Schneck & Henderson, 1990). Writing, using a primitive grasp pattern, is difficult to master; therefore school-aged children using them often require intervention by an occupational therapist. The primitive grasp patterns that will be discussed in this text include the radial cross palmar grasp, palmar supinate, digital pronate, brush grasp, and grasp with extended fingers (Table 5-1).

Transitional grasps are typically used as a child moves from the use of a primitive grasp pattern to a mature grasp pattern. These grasps are usually seen in children between 3 and 6 years of age (Schneck & Henderson, 1990). Transitional grasps include the static quadrupod, cross thumb, and the static tripod grasp (see Table 5-1). These grasps continue to have movements that originate in the shoulder, but an increased amount of mobility is seen at the wrist and elbow with the forearm resting on the table. Intrinsic movements of the hand are not seen in transitional grasp patterns. Bergmann (1990) found that not all supposed transitional grasps are transitional. She documented that a small percentage (5%) of adults in her study used the cross thumb and the static tripod grasps rather than a mature grasp pattern.

Mature grasp patterns are characterized by dynamic wrist control and the use of intrinsic and extrinsic muscles of the hand, which facilitate coordinated distal finger control. A mature grasp pattern requires the ability to isolate the movements of the fingers individually, with minimal involvement of the upper extremity and trunk. Mature grasp patterns can occasionally be seen in children as young as 3 years of age but are commonly seen in children between 4 and 6 years of age (Schneck & Henderson, 1990). Bergmann (1990) found that 86% of nearly 500 adults used the dynamic tripod with another 10% using the lateral tripod. The lateral tripod, dynamic quadrupod, dynamic tripod, and the interdigital tripod are typically considered mature grasp patterns (see Table 5-1).

Five *additional pencil grasps* have been included to illustrate the numerous pencil grasp variations found in the literature and clinical practice.

Table 5-1

COMPARISON OF HANDWRITING GRASP NAMES BY AUTHOR

	Halverson, Thompson, Ilg, et al., 1940	McBride, 1942	Wynn-Parry, 1966	Sherik, Weiss, & Flatt, 1971	Rosen-bloom & Horton, 1971	Morrison, 1978	Saida & Miyashita, 1979	Kamakura, Matsuo, Ishii, Mitsuboshi, & Miura, 1980	Bergman, 1990
Radial Cross Palmar	Cross palmar					Cross palmar			
Palmar Supinate							Palmar grasp		
Digital Pronate					Pronate method		Pronate method		
Brush Grasp									
Grasp with Extended Fingers									
Static Quadrupod									
Cross Thumb									Cross thumb
Static Tripod					Tripod posture		Tripod posture		Static tripod
Lateral Tripod									Lateral tripod
Dynamic Quadrupod		Thumb-finger gtrip		Three-point palmar pinch					
Dynamic Tripod			Dynamic tripod		Dynamic tripod		Dynamic tripod	Tripod grip	Dynamic tripod
Interdigital Tripod									

Comparison of Handwriting Grasp Names by Author, continued

Table 5-1

	Schneck & Henderson, 1990; and Schneck, 1991	Myers, 1992	Hanft & Marsh, 1993	Erhardt, 1994	Amundson, 1995	Benbow, 1995	Amundson, 1998	Bruni, 1998	Peterson, 1999	Dennis & Swinth, 2001	Summers, 2001	Benbow, 2002
Radial Cross Palmar	Radial cross palmar											
Palmar Supinate	Palmar supinate			Palmar supinate				Palmar supinate		Palmar supinate		
Digital Pronate	Digital pronate			Digital pronate				Digital pronate and Radial palmar		Digital pronate		
Brush Grasp	Brush grasp											
Grasp with Extended Fingers	Grasp with extended fingers											
Static Quadrupod		Static quadripod				Quadrupod					Static quadrupod	Static quadrupod
Cross Thumb	Cross thumb				Cross thumb							
Static Tripod	Static tripod			Static tripod posture	Static tripod			Immature & Static tripod		Static tripod		Static tripod
Lateral Tripod	Lateral tripod	Lateral tripod			Lateral tripod	Lateral tripod				Lateral tripod	Lateral tripod	
Dynamic Quadrupod	Four finger	Dynamic quadripod			Four finger & Quadrapod	Quadrupod				Quadropod	Dynamic quadrupod	Dynamic quadrupod
Dynamic Tripod	Dynamic tripod	Dynamic tripod	Dynamic tripod	Dynamic tripod posture	Dynamic tripod	Dynamic tripod	Dynamic tripod	Dynamic tripod	Dynamic Tripod	Dynamic tripod	Dynamic tripod	Dynamic tripod
Interdigital Tripod						Adapted tripod	Monk's grasp					Adapted tripod

Pictorial Summary of Handwriting Grasps

Primitive Handwriting Grasps . . . .

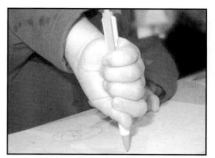
Radial Cross Palmar
Grasp, pg. 64

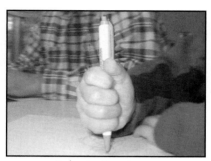
Palmar Supinate
Grasp, pg. 65

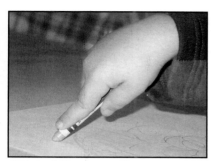
Digital Pronate Grasp, pg. 66

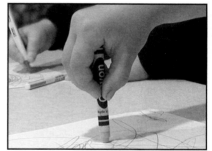
Brush Grasp, pg. 67

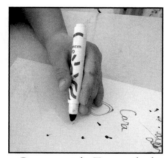
Grasp with Extended
Fingers, pg. 68

Transitional Handwriting Grasps . . . .

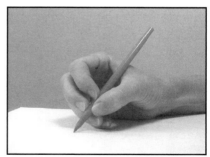
Static Quadrupod Grasp,
pg. 70

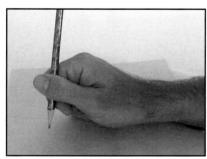
Cross Thumb Grasp, pg. 71

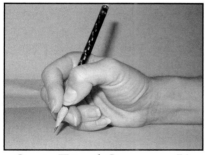
Static Tripod Grasp, pg. 72

Pictorial Summary of Handwriting Grasps

Mature Handwriting Grasps . . . .

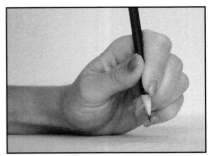

Lateral Tripod Grasp, pg. 74

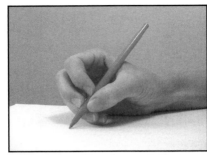

Dynamic Quadrupod Grasp, pg. 75

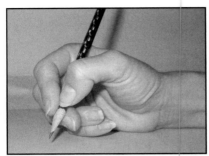

Dynamic Tripod Grasp, pg. 76

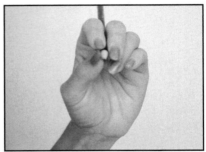

Interdigital Tripod Grasp, pg. 77

Additional Pencil Grasps . . . .

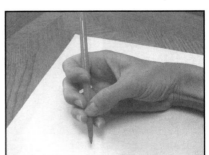

Index Grip, pg. 78

PRIMITIVE GRASP PATTERNS

RADIAL CROSS PALMAR GRASP

(Schneck & Henderson, 1990; Schneck, 1991)

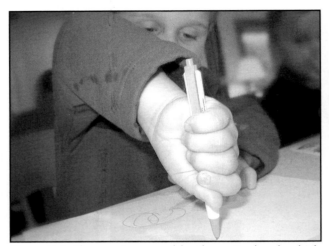

Figure 5-1. The pen is grasped by the entire hand, which does not allow the precise hand and finger movements needed for mature writing. Observe that the forearm does not rest on the table.

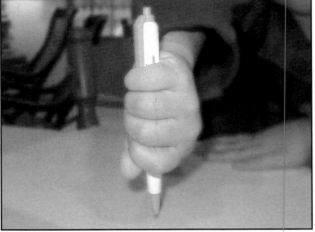

Figure 5-2. This grasp is much like the palmar supinate, but differs in that the forearm in the radial cross palmar is held in pronation.

Alternative Grasp Name

- *Cross Palmar Grasp* (Halverson, Thompson, Ilg, et al., 1940; Morrison, 1978)

Description of the Hand

The pencil or crayon is positioned in a fisted hand with the tip of the instrument projecting out from between the thumb and index finger. The thumb is positioned on the radial side of the index finger.

Description of the Wrist, Forearm, and Arm

The wrist ranges from slight flexion to extension with ulnar deviation, while the forearm is pronated. The arm is not supported on the table when drawing. Lateral movements of the shoulder (Halverson et al., 1940; Morrison, 1978) produce full arm movements (Schneck & Henderson, 1990; Schneck, 1991) that control the pencil or crayon.

Interesting Information

In their 1940 study, Halverson et al. reported that a child raises his hand high and often misses the paper when attempting to color. This may be the first pencil grasp that is used by a child. This grasp is usually seen in children around 1 year of age.

PALMAR SUPINATE GRASP

(Schneck & Henderson, 1990; Schneck, 1991; Erhardt, 1994; Bruni, 1998; Dennis & Swinth, 2001)

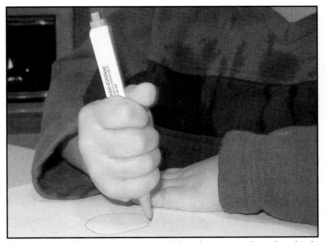

Figure 5-3. The pen is grasped by the entire hand, which does not allow the precise hand and finger movements needed for writing.

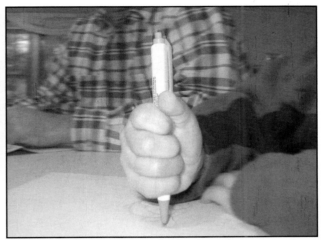

Figure 5-4. This grasp is much like the radial cross palmar, but differs in that the forearm in the palmar supinate is held in a more neutral position.

Alternative Grasp Name

- *Palmar Grasp* (Saida & Miyashita, 1979)

Description of the Hand

The crayon is held in a fisted hand, with the tip of the instrument extending from the ulnar side. The thumb is positioned on the radial side of the index finger.

Description of the Wrist, Forearm, and Arm

The wrist ranges from slight flexion to extension. The forearm is positioned in the neutral position (between pronation and supination). Full arm movements continue to dominate the drawing process, and the hand is not supported on the table.

Interesting Information

This grasp is typically seen in children around 1 to 1.5 years of age (Erhardt, 1994). The child using a primitive grasp at this age lacks the motor control of the hand and arm not only to grip the crayon in a precision grip, but also to draw vertical lines or color within the lines. "The first scribbles are actually angular zig-zag lines, which are related to the lever construction of the arm joints" (Erhardt, 1992, p. 20).

The radial cross palmar and the palmar supinate grasp differ in the position of the forearm and the position of the pencil tip. In the radial cross palmar, the forearm is pronated, while in the palmar supinate, the forearm is closer to a neutral position. The grasp changes as the forearm position matures and changes. The forearm is positioned in pronation during the child's first reaching pattern. As the child matures, the forearm position is more neutral during reach and grasp. In both of the aforementioned grasps, the pencil movement continues to be controlled by the shoulder, as the arm is still functioning as one unit (Conner et al., 1978).

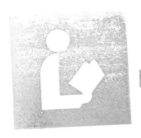

DIGITAL PRONATE GRASP

(Schneck & Henderson, 1990; Schneck, 1991; Erhardt, 1994; Bruni, 1998; Dennis & Swinth, 2001)

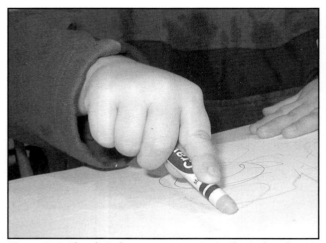

Figure 5-5. The digital pronate grasp is similar in hand position to the diagonal volar grasp, but since the functions are fundamentally different it is classified separately.

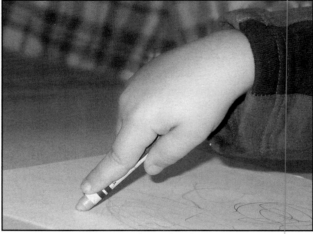

Figure 5-6. 5-6 Note that the index finger is extended along the shaft of the pencil, thereby providing greater precision in this still primitive grasp.

Alternative Grasp Names

- *Radial Palmar* (Bruni, 1998)
- *Pronate Method* (Rosenbloom & Horton, 1971; Saida & Miyashita, 1979)

Description of the Hand

This grasp is characterized by the end of the pencil or crayon extending past the ulnar aspect of the palm. The index finger is extended along the shaft of the instrument toward the tip while the middle, ring, and little fingers are curled around the upper the crayon portion of or pencil.

The thumb is not opposed, but lies along the shaft of the pencil.

Description of the Wrist, Forearm, and Arm

The forearm is pronated with the wrist held in a neutral to slightly flexed position. The arm is not positioned on the table when writing (Morrison, 1978; Schneck & Henderson, 1990; Schneck, 1991). Full arm movements are used to draw while using this grasp (Schneck & Henderson, 1990; Schneck, 1991).

Interesting Information

This grasp is typically seen between the ages of 2 and 3 years (Dennis & Swinth, 2001). Saida and Miyashita (1979) hypothesize that this grasp is more likely to be seen in children who use forks and knives, due to the position of the hand when using a knife.

BRUSH GRASP

(Schneck & Henderson, 1990; Schneck, 1991)

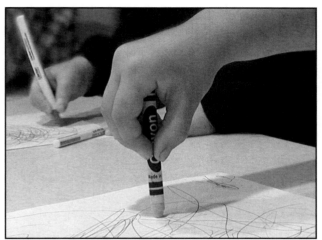

Figure 5-7. Notice the use of the arches and the thenar and hypothenar eminences to assist the fingers in securing the crayon in the palm while using the brush grasp. Note that the forearm does not rest on the table.

Description of the Hand

The eraser end of the pencil (or flat end of a new crayon) is secured in the palm with the pencil shaft held by the fingertips (Schneck & Henderson, 1990; Schneck, 1991). All PIP and DIP joints of the finger are positioned in slight flexion to full extension. MCP joints are flexed, as they surround the shaft of the pencil. The hypothenar eminence is important, due to the oblique direction of the little finger as it crosses the palm toward the pencil. The thumb is in beginning opposition. Both the longitudinal and transverse arches are active in this grasp. The longitudinal arch is aligning the MCP joints with the finger phalanges, and the transverse arches are positioning the MCP and carpal bones to allow the opposition of the thenar and hypothenar eminence.

Description of the Wrist, Forearm, and Arm

The pronated forearm is not supported on the table, as full arm movements move the pencil with the assistance of the flexed wrist (Schneck & Henderson, 1990; Schneck, 1991).

Interesting Information

The child continues to lack the ability to manipulate the pencil with the small, isolated finger movements required for mature writing. Therefore, the child will continue to use full arm movements until distal maturation develops.

GRASP WITH EXTENDED FINGERS

(Schneck & Henderson, 1990; Schneck, 1991)

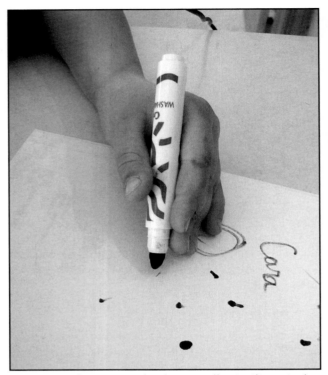

Figure 5-8. This grasp is developmentally significant in that the pencil is secured primarily with the radial fingers and thumb.

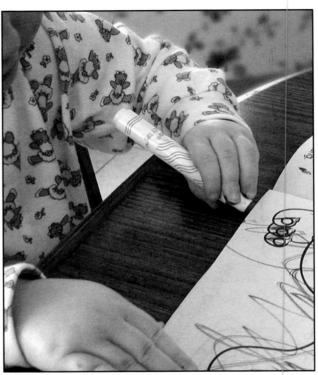

Figure 5-9. The ulnar fingers are not flexed into the palm to provide support. As a result, the grasp with extended fingers offers less stability to the radial side of the hand for intrinsic movements.

Description of the Hand

The pencil is held between the radial fingers and thumb, with the IP joints positioned in slight flexion to extension. The ulnar digits, if flexed, are not flexed into the palm. The thumb is beginning to oppose the fingers, an important skill for the development of a mature grasp pattern. The pencil is resting on the web space between the index finger and thumb.

Description of the Wrist, Forearm, and Arm

The wrist position varies from radial to ulnar deviation; the forearm is pronated as it moves as a unit to draw (Schneck & Henderson, 1990; Schneck, 1991).

Interesting Information

This grasp has less stability than a more mature grasp pattern due to the extension of the ulnar digits. The stability provided by the disassociation between the ulnar and radial sides of the hand, which is seen when the ulnar digits are flexed against the palm, remains undeveloped.

TRANSITIONAL GRASP PATTERNS

STATIC QUADRUPOD GRASP

(Myers, 1992; Summers, 2001; Benbow, 2002)

Alternative Grasp Name

- *Quadrupod Grasp* (Benbow, 1995)

Description of the Hand

This transitional grasp is characterized by the pencil being stabilized against the lateral side of the ring finger with the index and middle fingers placed on the pencil shaft. The thumb is opposed. The MCP and IP joints of the fingers are flexed to support the pencil. The little finger is flexed toward the palm for support and stabilization (Benbow, 2002). The pencil rests in the "partially to completely open web space" (Amundson, 1995, p. 44).

Description of the Wrist, Forearm, and Arm

The wrist is extended 25 to 35 degrees and the forearm is supinated 50 to 60 degrees from a fully pronated position (Benbow, 2002). The hand moves as a unit in this static grasp, with movement originating in the proximal upper extremity joints that reduces writing speed and refinement (Benbow 2002). The forearm is positioned on the desktop (Schneck & Henderson, 1990; Schneck, 1991).

Interesting Information

This grasp often moves from a static quadrupod to a dynamic quadrupod (Myers, 1992; Benbow 2002). The

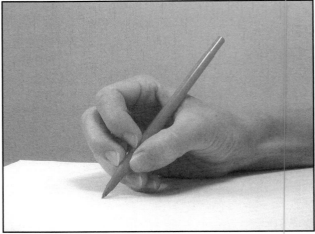

Figure 5-10. Notice the placement of two fingers on the shaft of the pencil with an opposing thumb in the static quadrupod grasp. The addition of the middle finger increases the stability of the pencil and differentiates this grasp from the static tripod.

transition to a dynamic grasp can be seen when the intrinsic muscles of the hand begin to move the pencil as opposed to the larger and more proximal muscles of the upper extremity. This shift is similar to the static and dynamic tripod grasps

CROSS THUMB GRASP

(Schneck & Henderson, 1990; Bergmann, 1990; Schneck, 1991; Amundson, 1995)

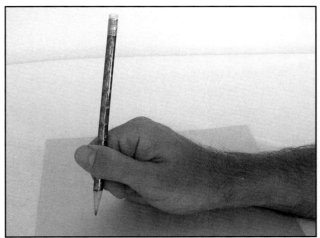

Figure 5-11. Note the differences in thumb position of these examples of the cross thumb grasp: this photo shows the shaft of the pencil secured by the pad of the thumb against the index finger.

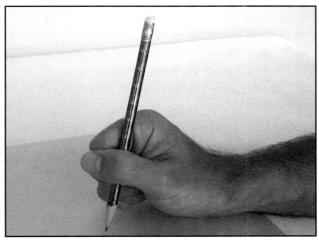

Figure 5-12. This photo is an example of the shaft of the pencil secured within a flexed IP joint.

Description of the Hand

This grasp is characterized by flexion of all of the fingers into the palm, with the pencil held against the radial side of the index finger. The thumb is crossed over the pencil toward the index finger (Schneck & Henderson, 1990; Schneck, 1991) or can be overlapping the index finger (Amundson, 1995). The thumb is not opposed, but rather adducted, suggesting that the three muscles of the thenar eminence are being substituted by the adductor pollicis (Benbow, 1995). The web space is partially to completely closed.

Description of the Wrist, Forearm, and Arm

The wrist and the flexed fingers move the pencil as the forearm rests on the table (Schneck & Henderson, 1990; Schneck, 1991).

Interesting Information

The adducted thumb closes the web space between the thumb and index finger. Summers (2001) noted that IP and MCP joint laxity of the thumb was frequently seen with the thumb positioned in adduction. With a closed web space, the proprioceptive feedback is decreased. This proprioceptive feedback plays a role in grading the fine motor muscles of the hand (Benbow, 1995).

STATIC TRIPOD GRASP

(Schneck & Henderson, 1990; Bergmann, 1990; Schneck, 1991; Amundson, 1995; Bruni, 1998; Dennis & Swinth, 2001; Benbow, 2002)

Alternative Grasp Names

- *Tripod Posture* (Rosenbloom & Horton, 1971; Saida & Miyashita, 1979)
- *Static Tripod Posture* (Erhardt, 1994)
- *Immature Tripod* (Bruni, 1998)

Description of the Hand

This grasp is typically identified as a transitional grasp. The static tripod grasp shares the same hand position as the dynamic tripod, but the static tripod lacks the intrinsic hand movements typically seen in the dynamic tripod grasp (Rosenbloom & Horton, 1971). This tripod posture or static tripod grasp is characterized by the opposition of the pad of the thumb and the pad of the index finger, with the pencil secured between them while resting in the open web space between the two. The pencil is resting against the radial border of the middle finger on or near the distal phalanx. The longitudinal arch and transverse arches support the tripod posture. The fourth and fifth fingers are flexed into the palm, increasing the stability of the transverse metacarpal arch, and shifting control to the radial side of the hand (Benbow, 2002). As the static tripod develops, finger placement on the pencil moves toward the distal end of the pencil (Rosenbloom & Horton, 1971). This position provides the stability to enable the eventual distal intrinsic movement of the dynamic tripod (Rosenbloom & Horton, 1971).

Description of the Wrist, Forearm, and Arm

"The wrist is stabilized in about 20 degrees of extension" (Benbow, 2002, pg.265). The hand moves as a unit

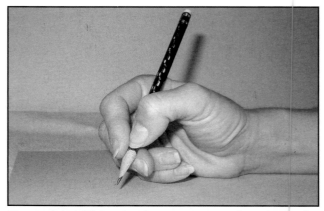

Figure 5-13. This tripod posture is used in both the dynamic and the static tripod grasps. The static tripod uses the wrist and hand as a unit to move the pencil, which differentiates this grasp from the dynamic tripod.

with additional mobility at the elbow and wrist but it now rests on the table with less movement from the shoulder.

Interesting Information

This grasp is typically seen in a 3- to 4-year-old child (Dennis & Swinth, 2001). This developmental progression from the static to the dynamic tripod grasp is characterized by the breaking up of gross motor movement patterns of the static tripod into finer, more selective, and intricate patterns that are characteristic of the dynamic tripod grasp (Conner et al., 1978).

MATURE GRASP PATTERNS

LATERAL TRIPOD GRASP

(Schneck & Henderson, 1990; Bergmann, 1990; Schneck, 1991; Myers, 1992; Amundson, 1995; Benbow, 1995; Dennis & Swinth, 2001; Summers, 2001)

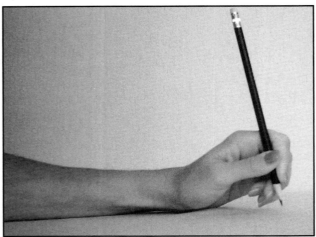

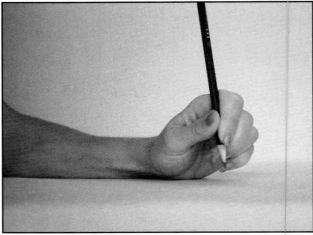

Figure 5-14. Note the relatively closed web space caused by the adducted thumb. This position limits the intrinsic movements while using this lateral tripod grasp.

Figure 5-15. This grasp is considered a lateral tripod grasp because the thumb is not in full opposition to the index and middle fingers. This grasp is differentiated from the dynamic tripod grasp in which the thumb is fully opposed.

Description of the Hand

This grasp is characterized by the stabilization of the pencil against the radial side of the middle finger with the volar surface (PIP to the fingertip pad) of the index finger placed on top of the shaft of the pencil. The thumb is adducted over the pencil and is placed anywhere along the index finger. The web space between the thumb and index finger is "partially to completely closed" (Amundson, 1995, p. 44). The 4th and 5th digits are flexed to provide stabilization of the transverse metacarpal arch and the middle finger (Schneck & Henderson, 1990; Schneck, 1991). The wrist and the PIP and MCP joints of the fingers (not the thumb) control the pencil (Summers, 2001).

Description of the Wrist, Forearm, and Arm

The wrist is slightly extended, with movement originating in the three radial digits with wrist movements tak-

ing part on tall and horizontal strokes (Schneck & Henderson, 1990). The forearm rests on the desktop.

Interesting Information

The increased surface contact between the fingers and the pencil shaft may indicate "a need for increased stabilization of the pencil and may result in less intrinsic muscular use during writing" (Dennis & Swinth, 2001, p. 181). Although the dynamic tripod grasp has historically been the considered the ideal pencil grasp, the lateral tripod grasp is a commonly used grasp pattern among children and adults. Schneck and Henderson (1990) found that 25% of 320 6-year-olds used the grasp, and Bergmann (1990) found that 10% of nearly 500 adults used it as well.

DYNAMIC QUADRUPOD GRASP

(Myers, 1992; Summers, 2001; Benbow, 2002)

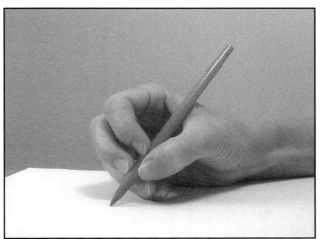

Figure 5-16. Notice the placement two fingers on the shaft of the pencil with an opposing thumb in the dynamic quadrupod grasp. This posture is identical to the static quadrupod grasp. However, the dynamic quadrupod grasp uses intrinsic movements to control the pencil.

Alternative Grasp Names

- *Quadrupod Grasp* (Amundson, 1995; Benbow, 1995; Dennis & Swinth, 2001)
- *Four Finger Grasp* (Schneck & Henderson, 1990; Schneck, 1991; Amundson, 1995)

Description of the Hand

This mature grasp is characterized by the pencil being stabilized against the lateral side of the ring finger with the index and middle fingers placed on the pencil shaft. The thumb is opposed to the two radial fingers on the pencil. The MCP and IP joints of the fingers are flexed. The little finger is flexed toward the palm for support and stabilization (Benbow, 2002). The pencil rests in the "partially to completely open web space" (Amundson, 1995, p. 44). The position of the pencil held in the hand is identical to the static quadrupod grasp, however the intrinsic muscles play a role in moving the pencil in the dynamic quadrupod.

Description of the Wrist, Forearm, and Arm

The wrist is extended 25 to 35 degrees and the forearm is supinated 50 to 60 degrees from a fully pronated position (Benbow, 2002). The forearm is positioned on the desktop (Schneck & Henderson, 1990; Schneck, 1991).

Interesting Information

This is considered to be an efficient pencil grasp (Benbow, 2002). "The additional fingers on the pencil adds power" (Benbow, 1995, p. 267) and also provides increased surface contact between the fingers and the pencil shaft. The quadrupod grasp may be used to counterbalance laxity in the index finger (Summers, 2001), using the middle finger to increase stabilization of the pencil (Benbow, 1995). Summers (2001) proposed that the position of the middle finger on the pencil shaft might help reduce the force on the flexor muscles of the index finger by distributing the load across the two fingers.

DYNAMIC TRIPOD GRASP

(Wynn-Parry, 1966; Rosenbloom & Horton, 1971; Saida & Miyashita, 1979; Schneck & Henderson, 1990; Bergmann, 1990; Schneck, 1991; Myers, 1992; Hanft & Marsh, 1993; Amundson, 1995; Benbow, 1995; Amundson, 1998; Bruni, 1998; Peterson, 1999; Dennis & Swinth, 2001; Summers, 2001; Benbow, 2002)

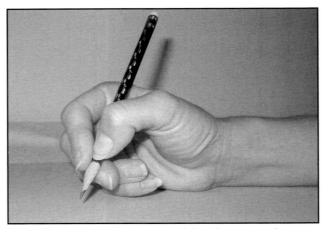

Figure 5-17. Observe the opposed thumb, open web space, and the clear differentiation of ulnar and radial sides of the hand which creates the tripod posture seen in the dynamic and static tripod grasps. The dynamic tripod grasp uses intrinsic musculature to move the pencil.

Alternative Grasp Names

- *Thumb-Finger Grip* (McBride, 1942)
- *Pen Grip* (Jacobson & Sperling, 1976)
- *Writing Grip* (Jacobson & Sperling, 1976)
- *Precision Grip* (Jacobson & Sperling, 1976)
- *Finger Tip Grip* (Jacobson & Sperling, 1976)
- *Three Fingers* (Jacobson & Sperling, 1976)
- *Three Point Palmar Pinch* (Sherik, Weiss, & Flatt, 1971)
- *Tripod Grip* (Kamakura, Matsuo, Ishii, Mitsuboshi, & Miura, 1980)
- *Dynamic Tripod Posture* (Erhardt, 1994)

Description of the Hand

The dynamic tripod grasp is characterized by the pencil being stabilized against the radial side of the distal phalanx of the middle finger while it is held between the pulps of the opposed thumb and index finger. The MCP and IP joints of the thumb, index, and middle fingers are flexed. The DIP of the index finger may be extended. The pencil rests in the rounded web space between the thumb and index finger, using a relaxed longitudinal arch. The fourth and fifth digits are flexed to stabilize the longitudinal arch and middle finger (Schneck & Henderson, 1990; Schneck 1991). The position of the pencil held in the hand is identical to the static tripod grasp, however the intrinsic muscles move the pencil in the dynamic tripod. The simultaneous flexion and extension of the tripod, especially at the IP joints, move the pencil in a proximal-distal axis (Elliott & Connolly, 1984). Yet, this pattern may be supplemented by a lateral deviation of the fingers, providing movement along the radial-ulnar axis (Schneck, 1991). The dynamic tripod grasp is thought to be the most efficient and skilled pencil grasp due to these intrinsic movements.

Description of the Wrist, Forearm, and Arm

The wrist is slightly extended and the forearm is resting on the table. The forearm is in more than 45 degrees of supination (from a fully pronated position) (Ziviani & Elkins, 1986).

Interesting Information

The dynamic tripod grasp can occasionally be seen in children as young as 3, but is seen on a more consistent basis in 4-year-olds (Schneck & Henderson, 1990). Yet once the pattern is developed, it continues to mature. Goodgold (1983) noted that kindergartners performed significantly better on handwriting tasks than pre-kindergarteners, indicating "that with maturity and experience, handwriting movement quality improves" (p. 473). Ziviani has studied the dynamic tripod grasp and its changes in 7- to 14-year-olds; noting that the grasp continues to develop through the 14th year (1982, 1983). Ziviani noted that younger children often have "more than 90 degrees of flexion of the PIP and hyperextension of the DIP with less than 45 degrees of forearm supination" (Ziviani, 1983, p. 780). Goodgold (1983) found that 80% of young children between the ages of 3.5 to 7.5 hold their pencils too tightly, thereby increasing the pressure on the joints. Ziviani (1983) and Goodgold (1983) go on to state that as these children mature, relaxation of the pencil grip is common. Supination tended to increase with age and was seen with the relaxation of the index finger (Ziviani, 1983). Ziviani (1982) hypothesized, based on her observation, that this pattern of relaxation may be a result of "the transition from print script to cursive writing" (p. 307).

INTERDIGITAL TRIPOD GRASP

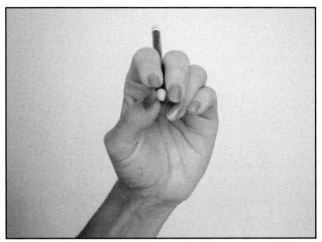

Figure 5-18. Note the similarity in hand position with that of the static or dynamic tripod. This grasp differs mainly in the placement of the writing utensil.

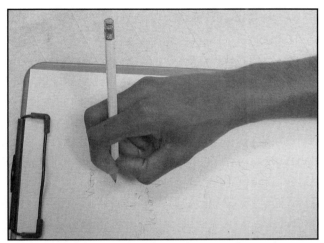

Figure 5-19. The interdigital tripod grasp relieves the stress placed on the MCP of the thumb in other tripod grasps.

Alternative Grasp Names

- *Adapted Tripod Grip* (Benbow, 1995; Benbow, 2002)
- *Monk's Grasp* (Amundson, 1998)

Description of the Hand

This grasp is characterized by the pencil resting in the second web space (between the index and middle finger), rather than the web space between the thumb and index finger. The pencil also rests on the radial side of the distal phalanx of the middle finger, with the index finger and thumb positioned on the pencil shaft. The two ulnar digits are flexed toward the palm. The MCP and PIP joints of the index finger are flexed with the DIP in slight flexion to extension. All joints of the middle finger are flexed. Pencil movement originates with simultaneous short flexion and extension patterns of the tripod. This grasp uses the same skilled muscles as the dynamic tripod grasp (Benbow, 1995).

Description of the Wrist, Forearm, and Arm

The wrist can vary from slight flexion to slight extension. The forearm is held in slight supination (from a fully pronated position).

Interesting Information

This grasp is a good alternative to other grasps due to the minimal amount of stress on the MCP joint of the thumb (Benbow, 1995). It is commonly recommended for individuals with arthritis or MCP joint pain in the thumb. Adults can usually make a smooth transition when adopting this grasp (Otto, Rarick, Armstrong, & Koepke, 1966), as "it is the most readily acceptable alternative grip when a child or an adult is having motor or orthopedic writing problems" (Benbow, 1995, p. 267).

ADDITIONAL PENCIL GRASPS

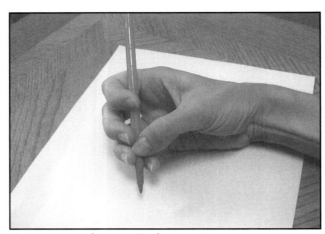

Figure 5-20. Index grip (Benbow, 2002).

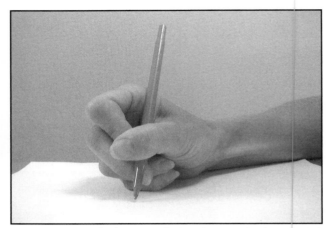

Figure 5-21. "Locked" grip with thumb wrap (Benbow, 2002).

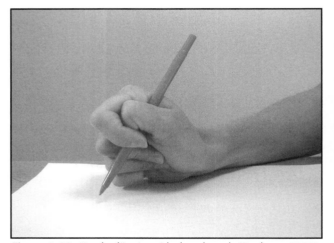

Figure 5-22. "Locked" grip with thumb tuck (Benbow, 2002).

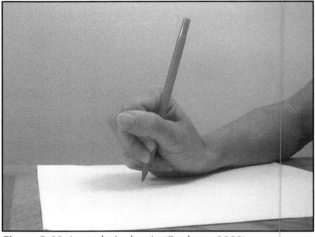

Figure 5-23. Lateral pinch grip (Benbow, 2002).

These additional pencil grasps have been included to provide a sense of the numerous variations of pencil grasps found in the literature and in clinical practice.

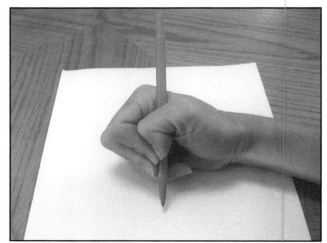

Figure 5-24. Lateral quadrupod grasp (Summers, 2001).

CHAPTER SIX

FUNCTIONAL HAND GRASPS

"It is in the human hand that we have the consummation of all perfection as an instrument" (Bell, 1834, p. 157). The hand is a remarkably complex, compact, intricate, and yet quiet piece of our anatomy that we use every minute of every day and often take for granted. It is an important mechanism that allows us to individualize our lives. The hand allows us to grasp; and using grasps we can do a myriad of things with our hands—ranging from expressing our deepest emotions, to accomplishing tasks at work, play and leisure, and holding multitudes of objects in as many ways.

This chapter is a compilation of selected photos, descriptions, information, and research about the hand and how we use it to grasp in activities of our daily lives. To organize these grasps, Napier's taxonomy of grasps was applied to divide them into power and precision grasps. Napier's landmark work on power and precision grasps has been regarded as one of the foremost contributions to "biological thinking" (Wilson, 1998, p. 129). According to Napier, a precision grasp is demonstrated when the distal pads of the opposed thumb and the pads of the fingertips are used. Large objects require that all the fingertips are used, but the smaller sized objects require only the thumb, index, and middle fingers. A power grasp is exhibited when the surface of the fingers and the palm contact the object and the thumb acts as an agent that reinforces.

Sometimes the thumb will guide the direction of the grasp. There can be precise movement even with a power grasp, as well as powerful movements with the precision grasp. Because not every grasp fits neatly within these divisions, we further divided these grasps into miscellaneous grasps, combination grasps that are both power and precision, and nonprehensile movements. The grasps are also alphabetized for easier referencing. Each grasp has the following sections: name, authors, source, description, overview of muscles, some interesting information, and functional uses (Tables 6-1, 6-2, 6-3, and 6-4).

Several grasps in this chapter have the same name in the developmental section. One of these grasps is the palmar grasp. Although this grasp has the same name and a similar description in both the functional and developmental sections, the palmar grasp is significantly different in the developing hand compared to the adult hand. For example, when compared to the developing hand the adult hand is larger, has more neurologic experience, and also has the capability to perform a variety of grasps from which the person can choose. In contrast, the developing child's hand has matured neither neurologically nor experientially and consequently has a limited repertoire of grasps it is capable of performing. Therefore, when a child uses a palmar grasp to secure a small object, that child is using the most precise grasp he or she is developmentally

Table 6-1

COMPARISON OF COMBINATION POWER
AND PRECISION GRASP NAMES BY AUTHOR

	Kamakura, Matsuo, Ishii, Mitsuboshi, & Miura, 1980	Moss & Hogg, 1981	Myers, 1992	Exner, 2001
Diagonal Volar	Power grip and Index finger extension		Diagonal volar	Power grasp
Ventral Grasp		Ventral grasp		

capable of using for that particular object. When a typically functioning adult hand uses a palm grasp he or she is likely using it because it works best for the particular situation, even though the hand is fully capable of using an array of other grasps.

Additionally, a grasp may appear in both the developmental and functional sections with similar descriptions but different names. For example, the pincer grasp in the developmental section is very similar to the pad to pad grasp in the functional section. The rationale for naming these nearly identical grasps differently is that these grasps are referred to differently in the literature depending on whether the grasp is referring to a developing child or an adult.

Table 6-2

COMPARISON OF POWER GRASP NAMES BY AUTHOR

	Halverson, 1931	Castner, 1932	Long, Conrad, Hall, & Furler, 1970	Weiss & Flatt, 1971	Sherik, Weiss, & Flatt, 1971	Connolly & Elliott, 1972	Connolly, 1973	Ammon & Etzel, 1977	Kamakura, Matsuo, Ishii, Mitsuboshi, & Miura, 1980	Moss & Hogg, 1981	Hogg & Moss, 1983
Cylindrical Grasp				Cylindrical grasp							
Hammer Grasp			Hammer grasp		Power grasp				Power grip standard Type		
Oblique Palmar Grasp						Oblique palmar				Oblique palmar	
Opposed Palmar Grasp							Opposed palmar			Opposed palmar	
Palmar Grasp	Palm and Hand grasp	Palmar prehension						Palmar grasp			
Reverse Transverse Palmar Grasp										Reverse transverse palmar	Reverse transverse palmar
Ring Grasp										Ring grasp	
Spherical Grasp				Spherical grasp					Surrounding mild flexion grip		

COMPARISON OF POWER GRASP NAMES BY AUTHOR, CONTINUED

Table 6-2

	Parks, 1988	Erhardt, 1994	Case-Smith, 1995	Duff, 1995	Edwards & Lafreniere, 1995	Provence, Erikson, Vater, & Palmeri, 1995	Belkin, English, Adler, & Pedretti, 1996	Bruni, 1998	Case-Smith & Bigsby, 2000	Exner, 2001
Cylindrical Grasp							Cylindrical grasp			Cylindrical grasp
Hammer Grasp										
Oblique Palmar Grasp										
Opposed Palmar Grasp										
Palmar Grasp	Palmar grasp	Palmar grasp	Palmar grasp	Palmar grasp		Palmar grasp		Palmar grasp	Palmar grasp	Palmar grasp
Reverse Transverse Palmar Grasp					Reverse transverse palmar					
Ring Grasp										
Spherical Grasp							Ball grasp			Spherical grasp

Table 6-3

Comparison of Precision Grasp Names by Author

	Halverson, 1931	Castner, 1932	Weiss & Flatt, 1971	Sherik, Weiss, & Flatt, 1971	Connolly & Elliott, 1972; & Connolly, 1973	Gesell & Amatruda, 1974	Ammon & Etzel, 1977	Conner, Williamson, & Siepp, 1978	Kamakura Matsuo, Ishii, Mitsuboshi, & Miura, 1980	Moss & Hogg, 1981
Disc Grasp			Disc grasp							
Dynamic Lateral Tripod Grasp									Tripod variation I	
Inferior Pincer Grasp								Inferior pincer		
Inferior Scissors Grasp						Radial raking				
Lateral Pinch									Lateral grip	
Pad to Pad		Pincer prehension	Standard palmar pinch		Adult 1972 and 1973	Inferior pincer			Tip prehension	Adult digital
Three Jaw Chuck	Forefinger grasp			Three point palmar pinch			Forefinger grasp			
Tip Pinch	Superior forefinger and Superior finger					Neat pincer grasp	Neat Pincer grasp			
Transverse Digital Grasp					Transverse digital, 1972					Transverse digital

Table 6-3

COMPARISON OF PRECISION GRASP NAMES BY AUTHOR, CONTINUED

	Newborg, Stock, Wnek, Guidubaldi, & Suinicki, 1984	Smith & Benge, 1985	Parks, 1988	Clarkson & Gilewich, 1989	Gilfoyle, Grady, & Moore, 1990	Johnson-Martin, Jens, Attermeier, & Hacker, 1991	Illingworth, 1991	Erhardt, 1994	Case-Smith, 1995	Duff, 1995
Disc Grasp										
Dynamic Lateral Tripod Grasp										
Inferior Pincer Grasp					Inferior pincer grasp	Inferior pincer grasp		Inferior pincer grasp		Inferior pincer grasp
Inferior Scissors Grasp			Raking grasp					Inferior scissors grasp		
Lateral Pinch				Lateral pinch	Lateral pinch					
Pad to Pad		Pad topad and Two point pinch			Superior pinch			Pincer grasp		Pincer grasp
Three Jaw Chuck		Three point pinch						3-jawed chuck		Three-jaw chuck
Tip Pinch	Neat pincer grasp		Neat pincer and Pincer		Prehension	Neat pincer grasp	Superior pincer grasp	Fine pincher	Superior pincer grasp	Superior pincer grasp
Transverse Digital Grasp										

Table 6-3

COMPARISON OF PRECISION GRASP NAMES BY AUTHOR, CONTINUED

	Provence, Erikson, Vater, & Palmeri, 1995	Trombly, 1995a	Belkin, English, Adler, & Pedretti, 1996	Bruni, 1998	Wilson, 1998	Case-Smith & Bigsby, 2000	Duff, Shumway-Cook, & Woollacott, 2001	Exner, 2001
Disc Grasp								Disc grasp
Dynamic Lateral Tripod Grasp								
Inferior Pincer Grasp				Inferior pincer grasp		Inferior pincer grasp		
Inferior Scissors Grasp								Crude raking grasp
Lateral Pinch							Key pinch	Lateral pinch
Pad to Pad						Superior pincer grasp		Pincer grasp
Three Jaw Chuck		Palmar pinch and Three jaw chuck	Palmar prehension		Three jawed chuck and Baseball grip			Three jaw chuck
Tip Pinch	Neat pincer grasp			Superior pinch and Pinch				Tip pinch
Transverse Digital Grasp								

Table 6-4   ## COMPARISON OF MISCELLANEOUS GRASP NAMES BY AUTHOR

	Napier, 1956 & 1993	Sherik, Weiss, & Flatt, 1971	Weiss & Flatt, 1971	Gesell & Amatruda, 1974	Kamakura, Matsuo, Ishii, Mitsuboshi, & Miura, 1980	Hogg & Moss, 1983	Parks, 1988	Myers, 1992	Erhardt, 1994	Tyldesley & Grieve, 1996	Wilson, 1998	Exner, 2001
Functional Scissors Grasp					Power grip (distal type)			Scissors grasp				
Hook Grasp	Hook grasp	Hook grasp	Hook grasp		Power grip- (hook type)							Hook grasp
Interdigital Grasp					Adduction grip	Inter- digital						
Lumbrical Grasp					Parallel extension grasp					Lumbrical and Plate grasp	Five-jawed cradle grip	
Raking Grasp				Radial raking			Raking grasp		Inferior scissors			Crude raking

PICTORIAL SUMMARY OF FUNCTIONAL GRASPS

Power Grasps . . . .

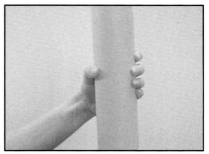

Cylindrical Grasp, pg. 92

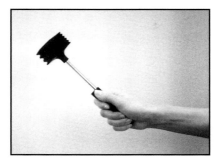

Hammer Grasp, pg. 94

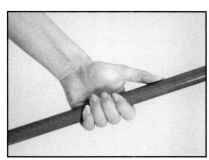

Oblique Palmar Grasp, pg. 95

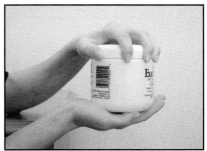

Opposed Palmar Grasp, pg. 96

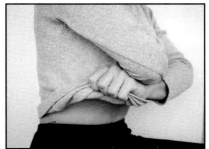

Palmar Grasp, pg. 97

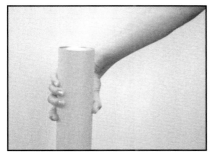

Reverse Transverse
Palmar Grasp, pg. 98

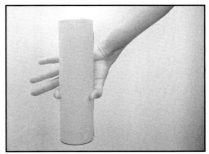

Ring Grasp, pg. 100

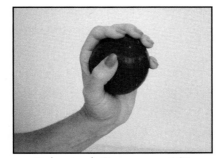

Spherical Grasp, pg. 101

Combination of Power and Precision Grasps . . . .

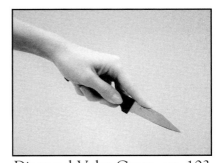

Diagonal Volar Grasp, pg. 103

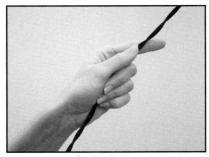

Ventral Grasp, pg. 104

Pictorial Summary of Functional Grasps

Precision Grasps. . . . .

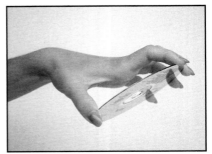

Disc Grasp, pg. 106

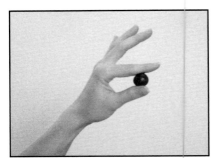

Dynamic Lateral Tripod
Grasp, pg. 108

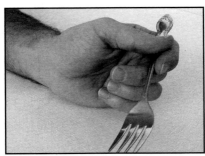

Inferior Pincer Grasp, pg. 110

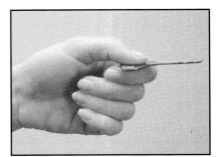

Lateral Grasp, pg. 111

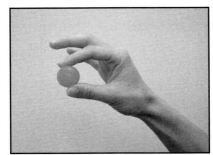

Pad to Pad Grasp, pg. 112

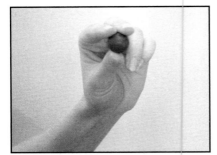

Three Jaw Chuck, pg. 114

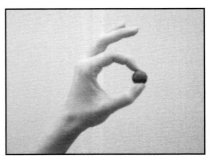

Tip Pinch, pg. 116

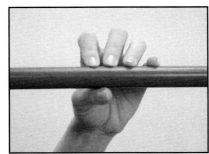

Transverse Digital Grasp,
pg. 118

PICTORIAL SUMMARY OF FUNCTIONAL GRASPS

Miscellaneous Grasps . . . .

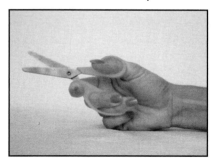

Functional Scissors Grasp, pg. 120

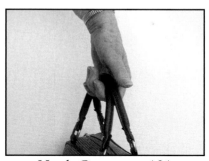

Hook Grasp, pg. 121

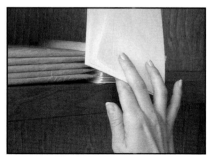

Interdigital Grasp, pg. 122

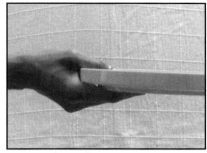

Lumbrical Grasp, pg. 123

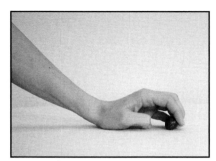

Raking Grasp, pg. 124

Nonprehensile Movements . . . .

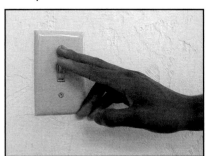

Pg. 125

POWER GRASPS

CYLINDRICAL GRASP

(Weiss & Flatt, 1971; Belkin, English, Adler, & Pedretti, 1996; Exner, 2001)

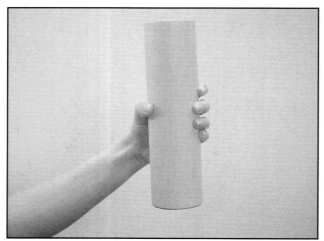

Figure 6-1. Observe the contact between the object and the palm of the hand. This involvement of the palm classifies this grasp as a power grasp.

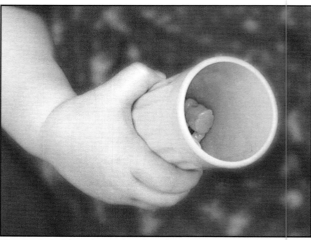

Figure 6-2. Note how the thumb acts as an opposing force to secure the object against the fingers and palm.

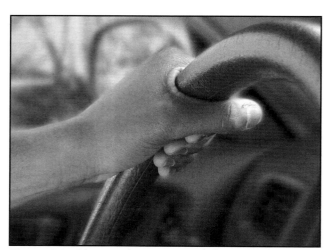

Figure 6-3. Observe the opening of the web space as it varies according to the size of the object relative to the hand.

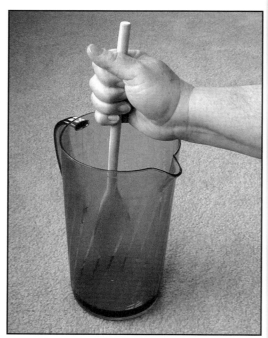

Figure 6-4. The active involvement of the thumb differentiates this grasp from the palmar grasp.

CYLINDRICAL GRASP, CONTINUED

(Weiss & Flatt, 1971; Belkin, English, Adler, & Pedretti, 1996; Exner, 2001)

Alternative Grasp Name

- *Transverse Palmar* (Moss & Hogg, 1981)

Description

In this grasp, the transverse arch is partially flattened and the longitudinal arch allows cupping of the object. The fingers are slightly abducted and have graded flexion of the IP and MCP joints. The palmar surface of the hand contacts the object when force is required (Weiss & Flatt, 1971). The thumb acts as an opposing force that allows the hand to grasp objects, such as a pot handle or the hand grasp used on a walker (Belkin et al., 1996). In this grasp, the wrist and forearm assume a variety of positions influencing the muscle balance and biomechanical features of the digital flexors. The person has the most strength in the digital flexors when the wrist is positioned in extension. Conversely, when the wrist is in flexion, the digital flexors are substantially weakened (Strickland, 1995).

Muscles

Both the extrinsic and intrinsic flexors and extensors of the fingers are required for use in this grasp. The thumb is positioned using the intrinsic musculature. Intrinsic and extrinsic muscles are used for thumb IP flexion or extension. If the intrinsic muscles are paralyzed, an imbalance of finger, arch, and thumb pressure will occur (Strickland, 1995).

Interesting Information

The cylindrical grasp is "the most common static grasp pattern" (Belkin et al., 1996, p. 327). Both hand size and length of the fingers will affect the strength of this grasp. The amount of pressure used during the grasp is modulated by a complex sensory system that signals the fingers, palm, and thumb to exert the correct amount of pressure in order to hold the object. If a person is missing the tactile sensibility to identify properties of an object, he or she will use proprioception. By using proprioception to compensate for tactile sensibility, the person can recognize the properties of the tool through a sense of force (Nakada & Uchida, 1997). Adequate sensory feedback is important for safety in order to prevent premature release or excess pressure (Tubiana et al., 1996). It has been hypothesized that this type of power grasp is evolutionarily millions of years old, having been used by our ancestors for power gripping of sticks and stones (Napier, 1993).

Functional Uses

Additional functional uses are holding a glass, a bicycle handle, a ladder, stabilizing a jar while the other hand twists a lid off, hanging on gym equipment, pushing a cart, and using cooking utensils.

HAMMER GRASP

Alternative Grasp Names

- *Hammer Squeeze* (Long et al., 1970)
- *Power Grasp* (Sherik et al., 1971)
- *Power Grip-Standard Type* (Kamakura et al., 1980)

Description

This grasp is characterized by stabilization of the object with the entire flexor surface of the palm, fingers, hypothenar eminence, and thumb. The thumb does not oppose the digits, but lies ventral to the object. Tightly adducted MCP joints and flexed IP joints of the fingers "hug" the object closely to the palm (Sherik et al., 1971). Flexion of the MCP joints of the fingers also help to bring the object into the palm for greater power and stability.

Muscles

The extrinsic flexors of the fingers curl around the object, while the thumb adductor and extrinsic and intrinsic thumb flexors provide the counterpressure needed to secure the object. The extrinsic thumb extensors not only position the thumb along the shaft of the object, but also provide some stability to the grasp. Long et al. (1970) conducted electromyographical studies of the activity in this type of grasp. They demonstrated that the first, second, and third dorsal interossei and the first and second palmar interossei are the active intrinsic muscles in this grasp. These interossei adduct the proximal phalanx to align them with the object, and then the extrinsic flexors can provide grasping power. The interossei provide a dual power role to the grasp because they also flex the MCP joints that provide more force to the grasp (Long et al., 1970).

Interesting Information

This grasp is keenly affected by the rich array of sensory and somatosensory mechanisms and dermatoglyphics of the hand. Together, these tactile and neurological mechanisms provide the person with the information to discern

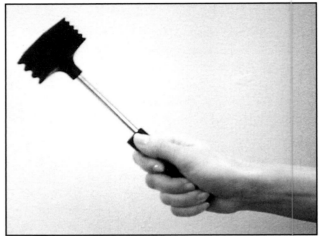

Figure 6-5. Note the surface contact of the whole hand against the object that enhances power and stability. The adduction of the thumb along the shaft of the object differentiates this grasp from the cylindrical grasp, in which the thumb is fully opposed to the fingers.

how much force is required to hold and release the object.

Several factors such as shape, size, and/or weight of the object impact hand and wrist position. Since the ring and little fingers flex more than 90 degrees in the hammer grasp, they can position themselves to make digito-palmar contact on the ulnar side of the hand and strengthen the grasp. These two ulnar fingers are only able to generate 70% of the force of the radial fingers. Consequentially, the hand relies on the radial digits for much of its power. Additionally, ulnar deviation of the wrist provides greater strength to this power grasp because it is in this position that the most force is generated at the phalanges (Hazelton, Smidt, Flatt, & Stephens, 1975).

Functional Uses

This grasp is used for grasping a hammer, drumsticks, paint brush, or holding an ax.

OBLIQUE PALMAR GRASP

(Connolly & Elliott, 1972; Moss & Hogg, 1981)

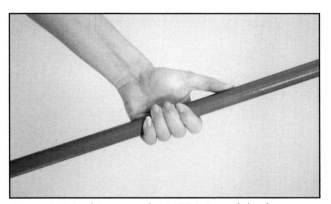

Figure 6-6. In this grasp, the MCP joints of the fingers are held in only slight flexion. This position allows the fingers to secure the object against the distal palm with the thumb acting as a stabilizer.

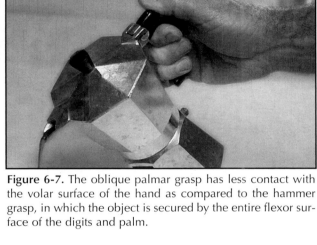

Figure 6-7. The oblique palmar grasp has less contact with the volar surface of the hand as compared to the hammer grasp, in which the object is secured by the entire flexor surface of the digits and palm.

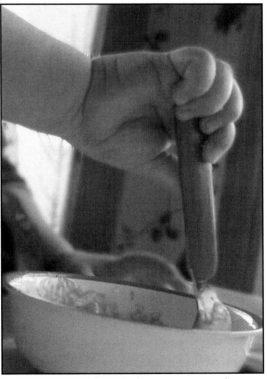

Figure 6-8. The oblique palmar grasp provides minimal power and stability. There-fore, this grasp may be used for activities requiring minimal power, such as eating with a utensil.

Description

In this grasp, the object lies obliquely across the palm and is secured to the palm with all the fingers. The thumb does not oppose the digits, but instead may lie ventral to the object (Connolly & Elliott, 1972). The thumb is used as a stabilizer in this grasp, which is one factor that distinguishes it from the otherwise similar hook grasp. It can be used for supporting, grasping, or manipulating an object.

Muscles

The extrinsic muscles are used to flex the fingers, along with the long thumb extensors that extend the IP and MCP joints of the thumb. Bendz (1980) concludes that simultaneous activity of both flexors and extensors occurs when the fingers make contact with an object and the grasp is secured.

Interesting Information

Although the fingers are different lengths when positioned in extension, when they are flexed around an object they appear to be of the same length. The differing lengths of fingers serve many purposes (Bell, 1834), such as allowing us to grasp a variety of sizes of spheres and oppose different fingers with a variety of force and position.

Functional Uses

This grasp can be used while holding a toothbrush to brush the teeth or when scooping pancakes with a spatula before flipping them.

Opposed Palmar Grasp

(Connolly, 1973; Moss & Hogg, 1981)

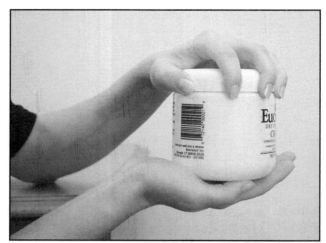

Figure 6-9. Note the abduction of the fingers and the flexion of the IP joints to accommodate the size of the object.

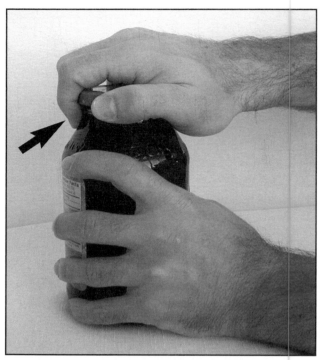

Figure 6-10. This grasp is considered a power grasp because of the palmar contact with the object. The opposed palmar grasp has a similar hand position to the disc grasp but, because the disc grasp contacts the object with only the fingers and thumb, it is classified as a precision grasp.

Description

The object is immobilized in the hand by being locked into the palm. The thumb is in an opposed position to the fingers with the object firmly held. No intrinsic movement is possible. This grasp is characterized as a power grasp because of the palmar and finger contact on the object. Note that the object may not contact the entire volar surface of the hand. The fingers are flexed primarily at the IP joints to grasp the object. In order to accommodate the object size, adaptation of this grasp takes place primarily at the CMC joint of the thumb and the MCP joints of the fingers (Strickland, 1995).

Muscles

The strength of the hand's extrinsic muscle flexors, as well as the wrist stabilizers, provide the power base for this grasp. The wrist is the "executive director" of the hand. First, it provides fine adjustments that position the hand for grasp. Then, it provides the stability for the fingers to grasp (Flatt, 1972). The wrist ligaments play a strategic role in stabilization. The thumb's position is accomplished by using the intrinsic and extrinsic abductors, as well as the thumb flexors.

Interesting Information

As the finger flexors need strength in this grasp, greater extension of the wrist will provide optimal lengthening for the long finger flexion and result in greater power to the finger flexors. The wrist is a key stabilizer in the complex movements required to grasp an object (Wells & Luttgens, 1976).

Functional Uses

This grasp is used for power action, such as opening tight lids on jars.

PALMAR GRASP

*(Ammon & Etzel, 1977; Parks, 1988; Erhardt, 1994; Case-Smith, 1995;
Duff, 1995; Provence et al., 1995; Bruni, 1998; Case-Smith & Bigsby, 2000; Exner, 2001)*

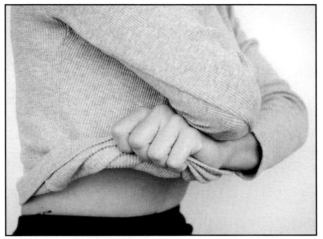

Figure 6-11. Notice that the thumb is acting as a stabilizer in this palmar grasp.

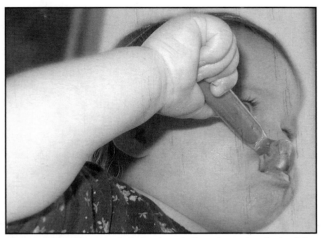

Figure 6-12. Observe that the thumb lies along the shaft of the spoon, while only the fingers press the object into the palm.

Alternative Grasp Names

- *Palm Grasp* (Halverson, 1931)
- *Hand Grasp* (Halverson, 1931)
- *Palmar Prehension* (Castner, 1932)

Description

The fingers are flexed at the MCP and IP joints to grasp the object. The thumb is positioned on the lateral aspect of the index finger and may be used to provide stabilization. The thumb may assume a passive rather than active role (Case-Smith, 1995).

Muscles

There is differentiation of the muscles on the ulnar and radial sides of the hand, with the object held predominately by the flexor extrinsics on the radial side. While all strong grasps require solidly intact median, radial, and ulnar nerves, this palmar grasp uses the radial side of the hand more than the ulnar side and therefore depends on the integrity of the median nerve.

Interesting Information

When a child uses a palmar grasp to secure a small object that child typically grasps the object in the middle of the palm, which is the most precise grasp he or she is developmentally capable of using. In contrast, an adult using a palmar grasp has developed the differentiation of the two sides of the hand, enabling him or her to grasp the object towards the radial side of the hand and use greater strength and precision.

Functional Uses

In the more mature hand, it is used functionally for dressing, such as pulling pants or underwear on or off or securing a towel while drying the back after a shower. It may also be used to grasp utensils for eating. Children commonly used this grasp to don and doff socks in a qualitative study of typically developing children (Buckland, McCoy, & Edwards, 1999).

REVERSE TRANSVERSE PALMAR GRASP

(Moss & Hogg, 1981; Hogg & Moss, 1983; Edwards & Lafreniere, 1995)

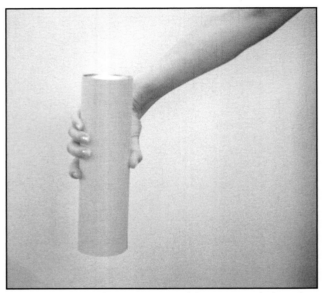

Figure 6-13. Notice the similarity of this grasp with the cylindrical grasp, with the differentiating factor being the pronated position of the forearm.

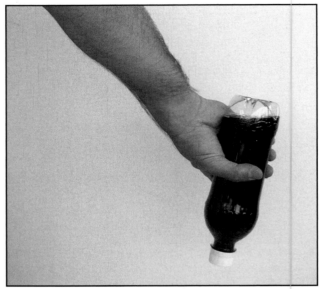

Figure 6-14. In this example of the reverse transverse palmar grasp, the wrist is in ulnar deviation to support the weight of the object.

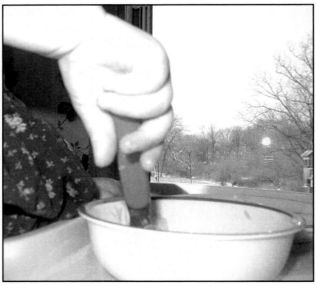

Figure 6-15. Note the variation in finger flexion depending on the size of the object.

Description

This grasp is similar to the cylindrical grasp because it uses the palm of the hand, fingers, and thumb to stabilize the object. The distinguishing factor of this grasp from the cylindrical grasp is the position of the forearm. In the reverse transverse palmar grasp, the forearm is pronated and the wrist is positioned in such a way that the palm faces away from the body (Hogg & Moss, 1983).

Muscles

This grasp requires the intrinsic and extrinsic muscles of the thumb and fingers, wrist flexors and extensors, and the pronators of the forearm. When the forearm is pronated, the wrist is more likely to access ulnar deviation to add power to a grasp.

Interesting Information

This grasp is observed in typically developing young children and older children with Down syndrome, as reported by Moss and Hogg (1981). The pronated position of the forearm and the extended elbow has a stabilizing effect that produces digital control. The child with Down syndrome may use this grasp to compensate for weak wrist action (caused by low muscle tone or anomalies of small or missing carpal bones) when using the sta-

REVERSE TRANSVERSE PALMAR GRASP, CONTINUED

(Moss & Hogg, 1981; Hogg & Moss, 1983; Edwards & Lafreniere, 1995)

bilization provided by the extended elbow and pronated forearm (Edwards & Lafreniere, 1995).

The reverse transverse palmar grasp, like other grasps, is dependent upon a fluid chain of joint movement to grasp an object. Int he typical hand, the sequence of digit flexion is PIP and MCP flexion followed by DIP flexion. If the sequence of flexion of phalanges is disrupted, it causes "diskinetic finger flexion or awkward function in grasp (Tubiana, et al., 1996).

Functional Uses

Children with Down syndrome may grasp a writing utensil or paint brush with a similar hand position, called a radial cross palmar. Because scribbling and grasping are fundamentally very different, these nearly identical hand positions are classified as separate grasps. Other uses for this grasp can be reaching behind the body for an object, or emptying a soda bottle or soup can.

RING GRASP

(Moss & Hogg, 1981)

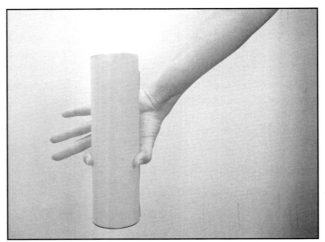

Figure 6-16. This grasp is differentiated from the reverse transverse palmer in the position of the ulnar digits and the lack of palmar contact on the ulnar side of the hand.

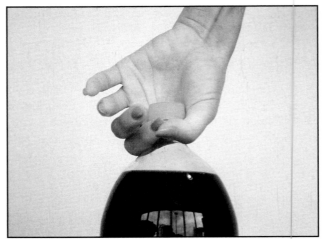

Figure 6-17. Observe the variation of the flexion and extension of the ulnar digits in the ring grasp.

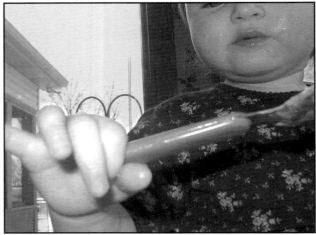

Figure 6-18. Note the different degrees of forearm pronation in the ring grasp.

Description

This grasp is similar to the reverse transverse palmar grasp, but uses only the index finger, thumb, and palm of the hand to secure the object. The forearm is in the same pronated position as the reverse transverse palmar grasp, and the hand is facing away from the body. The MCP and IP joints of the index and/or middle finger and thumb (as well as the longitudinal and transverse arches) will flex and extend to accommodate to the size of the object. The wrist may be positioned in neutral or ulnar deviation for increased power.

Muscles

The long index finger flexors and the long flexor of the IP joint of the thumb are used to position the finger(s) and thumb around the object. The first interossei, thumb intrinsics, and the wrist ulnar deviators provide the power and stability needed to secure the object.

Interesting Information

Ulnar deviation of the wrist exerts greater power than radial deviation. Therefore, when greater force is required, the wrist will ulnarly deviate to provide additional power.

Functional Uses

This grasp is used for emptying containers, carrying two-liter bottles, and using a salt or pepper shaker.

SPHERICAL GRASP

(Weiss & Flatt, 1971; Exner, 2001)

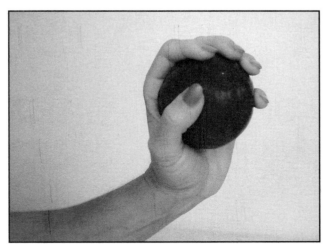

Figure 6-19. Notice the ulnar digits and their position relative to the radial side of the hand. This position of the ulnar digits provides the cupping of the object in the palm.

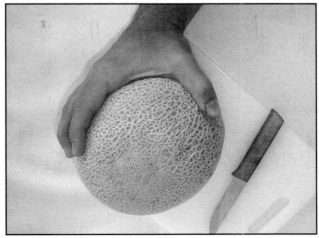

Figure 6-20. Note the accommodation of the web space according to the size of the object in the spherical grasp.

Alternative Grasp Names

- *Surrounding Mild Flexion Grip* (Kamakura et al., 1980)
- *Ball Grasp* (Belkin et al., 1996)

Description

Characteristics of the spherical grasp include stabilization of the wrist; abduction of the fingers; flexion at the MCP and IP joints; and stability of the longitudinal arch (Exner, 2001). "The hypothenar eminence lifts to assist the cupping of the hand for control of the object" (Exner, 2001, p. 296). The spherical grasp differs from the cylindrical grasp mainly in the positioning of the fourth and fifth digits. In the spherical grasp, the fourth and fifth digits assume a more flexed position that allows cupping of the palm. In the cylindrical grasp, the fourth and fifth digits are positioned in greater extension. Unlike the opposed palmar grasp, the spherical grasp demonstrates full contact of the volar (palmar) surface of the palm and digits. An intact power grasp usually has a distribution of pressure over the palmar surfaces of the hand, MCP heads, as well as the hypothenar and thenar eminences (Tubiana et al., 1996). The longitudinal arch assists the hand with flexion of the IP and MCP joints in this grasp, and provides flexibility by flattening and cupping the palm and fingers. This flexibility allows the person to pick up objects that vary in size (Duncan, 1989).

Muscles

This grasp requires the use of the extrinsic muscles to flex the IP joints of the fingers and the long thumb extrinsic muscle to flex the IP joint of the thumb to secure the object. The intrinsic muscles of the hand abduct the fingers and thumb to accommodate the size of the object.

Interesting Information

In 1834, Sir Bell asked the question, "Why are the fingers not of equal length?" If you grasp a ball, the points of fingers are equal! "This difference in length of fingers serves a thousand purposes,…" (p. 115). The different finger lengths give more variety and flexibility to hand grasps, including the ability to surround different sizes of spheres and shapes of objects.

In this grasp, the hypothenar eminence is important to opposition of the thumb and little finger (ulnar opposition). According to Wilson (1998, p. 30), "…the final biomechanical change at the base of the pinkie…" is quite remarkable and allows for ulnar opposition that significantly advanced the use of the hand. The best known of the earliest primates and (according to anthropologists and some theorists) a direct human ancestor is "Lucy," whose hand is estimated to be 3.2 million years old, could not use ulnar opposition (Wilson, 1998).

Functional Uses

This grasp can be used for turning a doorknob or holding a ball or any other round object.

COMBINATION OF POWER
AND PRECISION GRASPS

DIAGONAL VOLAR GRASP

(Myers, 1992)

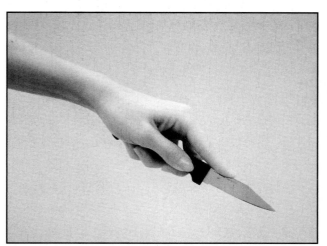

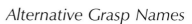

Figure 6-21. Note the use of the ulnar side of the hand to stabilize the object, and the extension of the index finger to provide more precise control over the object during an activity that requires both powerful and precise movements.

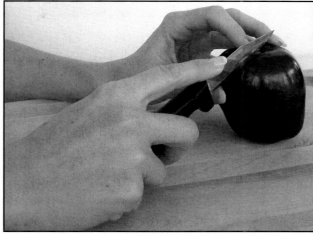

Figure 6-22. In the diagonal volar grasp, the extended index finger and thumb are used to guide the movement of the utensil, which differentiates it from the ventral grasp, in which the extended index finger and thumb are used to grasp the object.

Alternative Grasp Names

- *Power Grasp-Index Finger Extension Type* (Kamakura et al., 1980)
- *Power Grasp* (Exner, 2001)

Description

This is both a power and precision grasp where the object is stabilized by the ulnar side of the hand and directed by the pad of the extended index finger and thumb. The fingers on the ulnar side of the hand are flexed around the object. The tool is also counterbalanced and secured against the pad of the thumb and the palm of the hand. Strong wrist stabilization is imperative in this grasp.

Muscles

The extensor indicis and lumbricals, as well as the extensor digitorum, help position the index finger along the top of the shaft of the tool. The collateral ligaments assist with stabilizing the digits in extension. The long finger flexors position the remaining fingers in flexion. The intrinsics of the thumb are active for placement of the thumb in adduction or slight opposition. The biomechanical balance of the thumb extensor/flexor extrinsics provides the stable thumb position.

Interesting Information

This is an example of a combination power and precision grasp. It is also an example of the hand simultaneously combining finger extension and flexion. The sides of the hand separate into two motor functions; the ulnar side is flexed around the tool for maximum stability while the radial side is extended to direct the movement. This separation of the hand uses the counterbalance of the arch for holding the tool (Capener, 1956). This is referred to as the coupling action of the ulnar digits and functions in power grips and precision handling. If additional power is required when using this grasp, the wrist can supply it by using ulnar deviation.

Functions

This grasp can be used for cutting up foods, such as meat or potatoes; dicing vegetables; and precision cutting, such as cutting down the middle of an electrical cord.

Ventral Grasp

(Moss & Hogg, 1981)

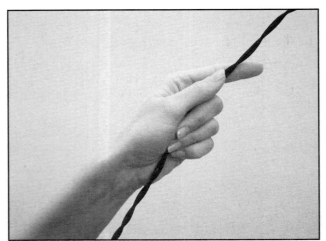

Figure 6-23. Note the use of the ulnar side of the hand to stabilize the object while the index finger and thumb grasp the object.

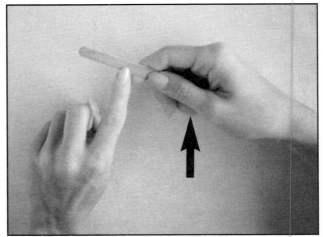

Figure 6-24. The grasp of the object with the index finger and thumb differentiate this grasp from the diagonal volar in which the extended index finger and thumb just guide the movement.

Description

This is a combined power and precision grasp, as defined by Napier (1956). This is because the object is secured by the palm and ulnar fingers, and simultaneously grasped by the extended to slightly flexed index finger and thumb. The thumb is adducted or opposed toward the lateral or ventral surface of the index finger.

Muscles

The extensor digitorum and lumbricals work together to stabilize the MCP joints and position the fingers in this grasp. The extrinsic flexor muscles of the middle, ring, and little fingers flex them against the palm. The extrinsic extensor muscles keep the index finger in a somewhat extended position. The thumb extrinsic extensors position the thumb in MCP and IP extension. The intrinsics of the thumb are active for placement of the thumb in adduction or slight opposition. When greater force is needed, the wrist will ulnarly deviate (Bendz, 1980) and the action of the lumbricals will be replaced by the stronger interossei.

Interesting Information

This grasp represents a disassociation of the sides of the hand, because the ulnar fingers are being used for stabilization and the radial fingers for grasping the objects. This is called coupling, as described by Capener (1956). The dissociation does not mean that the fingers or joints function completely independent of one another. In fact, "...no one single articulation in the hand is an isolated mechanical entity. Instead, each articulation functions as a part of a group arranged in kinetic chains" (Benbow, 1995, pg.257).

Functional Uses

This grasp serves to lock small, slippery, or thin objects (e.g., holding onto wire, string, or rope).

PRECISION GRASPS

Disc Grasp

(Weiss & Flatt, 1971; Exner, 2001)

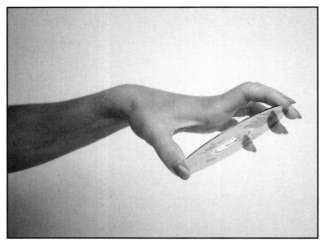

Figure 6-25. Observe the relative flatness of the arches of the hand holding the disc as opposed to the depth of the arches in the hand with a much smaller object.

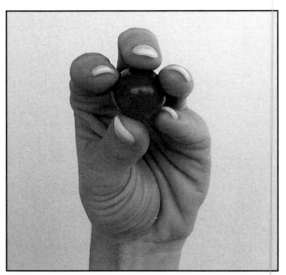

Figure 6-26. Note the abduction of the fingers and thumb depending on the size of the object.

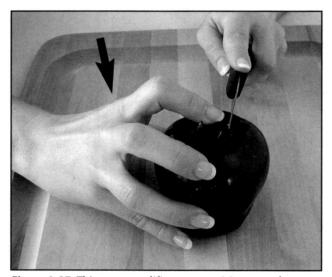

Figure 6-27. This grasp qualifies as a precision grasp because only the fingers and not the palm are engaged in grasping the object.

Description

The disc grasp is demonstrated when only the pads of the fingers make contact; the palm is not in contact with the object in this grasp. The fingers are flexed or extend-ed and abducted or adducted in a graded position to accommodate the size of the object. The CMC joint of the thumb and the MCP joints of the fingers are the primary joints that move to accommodate the size of the object (Strickland, 1995). The arches are more flattened with larger objects but they provide cupping of the hand in order to hold smaller objects.

Muscles

The long IP flexors of the thumb are active in this grasp. The long IP finger flexors, as well as ligament support, are important to provide the necessary alignment of the MCP and IP joints that influences the divergence or "spread finger" position of this grasp. The first and fourth dorsal interossei, the first and third palmar interossei, the fourth lumbrical, as well as the abductor digiti minimi muscles assist in providing finger abduction that is so characteristic of this grasp. Stabilization of the wrist is imperative.

The larger the object, the greater wrist movement and thumb extension is needed (Exner, 2001).

Interesting Information

The web space of the thumb provides full abduction of the thumb for grasp. The flexibility of the thumb's web

DISC GRASP, CONTINUED

(Weiss & Flatt, 1971; Exner, 2001)

space dictates the size of the object that can be grasped (Tubiana et al., 1996).

The grasp and manipulation of an object usually involves movement of the proximal joints of the hand. Individuals with impaired sensation often drop objects as soon as these joints are moved.

Functional Uses

This grasp is used to hold a small ball or to hold vegetables and fruits while cutting with the opposite hand.

DYNAMIC LATERAL TRIPOD GRASP

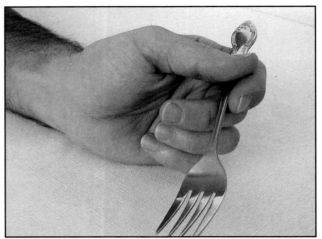

Figure 6-28. This grasp combines some characteristics of the lateral tripod (handwriting) grasp (i.e., the position of the index finger on the object and partial adduction of the thumb), but allows the small movements (flexion and extension of the PIP and DIP of the fingers) much like the dynamic tripod pencil grasp. That is one reason why the grasp is named the dynamic lateral tripod.

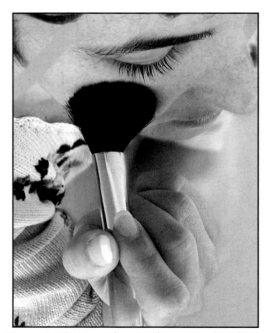

Figure 6-30. Note that in this example of the dynamic lateral tripod grasp, the thumb is in greater abduction than in the other examples.

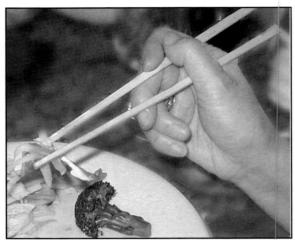

Figure 6-29. Note the similar hand position while using the chopsticks and the fork. Using chopsticks involves more movement of the IP joints as compared to using a fork.

Alternative Grasp Name

- *Tripod Variation I* (Kamakura et al., 1980)

Description

This grasp is characterized by an object held against the radial side of the middle finger near the DIP joint, with the pad of the index finger on top of the shaft of the tool. PIP joints are flexed, and DIP joints of the index and middle fingers range from moderate flexion to extension. All the fingers are flexed at the MCP joints; the ulnar fingers are flexed into the palm to give support to the metacarpal arch. The web space of the thumb is narrow, because the thumb is adducted or slightly opposed to secure the object against the radial border of the index finger. "This [hand position] is different from the Tripod Grip [dynamic tripod grasp], in that the thumb is more extended with adduction at the CMC joint. Often, MCP flexion of the ulnar fingers is slightly more than the Tripod Grip [dynamic tripod grasp]" (Kamakura et al., 1980, p. 441).

Muscles

The thumb adductor pollicis positions the thumb to secure the object, while thumb extrinsic flexors provide IP finger flexion. The lumbricals and interossei assist with the finger MCP flexion and the extrinsic flexors provide IP finger flexion.

DYNAMIC LATERAL TRIPOD GRASP, CONTINUED

Interesting Information

This grasp is used for eating with chop sticks, and it has been reported that Japanese children have more advanced prehension than children in other cultures—possibly as a result of using them (Saida & Miyashita, 1979). This grasp appears to be a precursor for the dynamic tripod grasp and assists in developing finger and thumb intrinsic muscles used in handwriting.

Both the longitudinal arch and transverse arches support the posture required for this grasp. The longitudinal arch supports the cupped shape of the hand in this grasp.

The relatively rigid transverse carpal arch provides the stability from which the distal structures can move. The transverse metacarpal arch is more mobile and assists with opposition of the thumb to the ulnar side of the hand. All of these arches are important in this grasp.

Functional Uses

This grasp is used for many different functional activities, including eating with a spoon or fork, using chopsticks, applying blush or lipstick, and knitting and crocheting.

INFERIOR PINCER GRASP

*(Conner et al., 1978; Gilfoyle et al., 1990; Johnson-Martin et al., 1991;
Erhardt, 1994; Duff, 1995; Bruni, 1998; Case-Smith & Bigsby, 2000)*

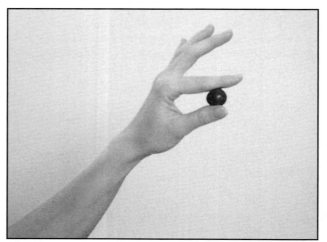

Figure 6-31. Note the position of the object proximal to the pad of the finger in the inferior pincer grasp.

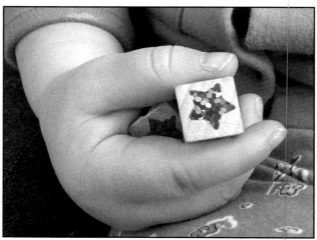

Figure 6-32. The position of the object in the inferior pincer grasp can be contrasted with the pad to pad grasp, where the object is secured between the pads of the fingers and thumb.

Description

This grasp requires isolation of the index finger and the thumb in opposition. The object is held between the ventral surface of the index finger, near the DIP joint, rather than at the tip or pad of the finger. The index finger is extended at the IP joints and flexed at the MCP joint. The thumb is also extended at the MCP and IP joints. The ulnar fingers may be extended for balance or flexed into the palm for support. The developing child also uses this grasp. However, because the typical adult has the neurological capability of full thumb opposition, the thumb adduction seen in the developing hand is not associated with the inferior pincer grasp in the adult hand.

Muscles

The lumbricals and interossei of the index finger provide flexion at the MCP joint, while allowing extension of the IP joints. The index finger is extended by the extensor indicis and extensor digitorum (Strickland, 1995). The extensor pollicis longus and brevis position the thumb in extension. The force for stabilizing the object is from the thumb intrinsics (opponens pollicis, abductor pollicis brevis, and flexor pollicis brevis). The adductor pollicis increases its contraction as more pressure is needed (Long et al., 1970).

Interesting Information

In order for true opposition to occur, several factors must be present in the thumb: adequate length, a saddle joint (the CMC), and the ability to rotate the thumb into opposition. The thumb supplies two indispensable components for grasp precision: stability and direction control (Duncan, 1998). These characteristics of the thumb earn it the designation of "24-karat thumb" (Wilson, 1998). The MCP joint of the thumb has the most flexibility; however, rotational movements in the index and other fingers must be present (Wilson, 1998).

As this grasp develops in the infant, the thumb moves from adduction to a more precise position of opposition. This grasp is developmentally significant for the infant because it is the beginning of thumb opposition.

Functional Uses

This grasp is important for in-hand manipulation skills, as it positions the hand for translation of objects or moving an object from palm-to-finger or finger-to-palm in the mature hand. This grasp is also used by children as they begin to hold food and other small objects.

LATERAL PINCH

(Clarkson & Gilewich, 1989; Gilfoyle et al., 1990; Exner, 2001)

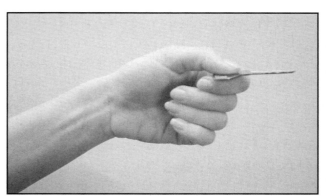

Figure 6-33. Note how the thumb flexors help to secure the object against the index finger.

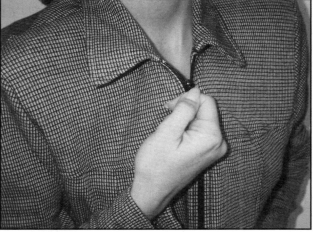

Figure 6-34. Because this grasp has partial opposition of the thumb, it is considered a precision grasp.

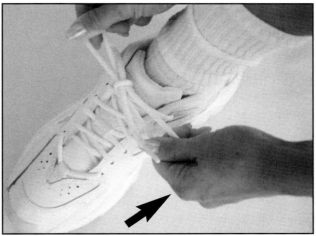

Figure 6-35. Notice that the thumb is neither fully opposed nor fully adducted.

Alternative Grasp Names

- *Lateral Grip* (Kamakura et al., 1980)
- *Key Pinch* (Duff et al., 2001)

Description

This frequently used grasp may be demonstrated by partial adduction or partial opposition, MCP and IP flexion, and slight CMC rotation of the thumb. Because the thumb CMC joint is in slight rotation, the thumb is not in a true adducted position. The thumb presses against the index finger to provide counterpressure (Clarkson & Gilewich, 1989). The pad of the thumb is typically positioned on the radial aspect of the flexed index finger at or near the DIP joint. The remaining fingers are held in flexion. The wrist stabilizes the other joints to allow more precision and pressure. The forearm and hand help to position the thumb so gravity can assist with adduction. This grasp provides less precision than the three jaw chuck, but has more power.

Muscles

The action of the first dorsal interosseous is very strong so the index finger can abduct and assist in stabilizing the object against the thumb. The flexor digitorum profundus and superficialis, along with intrinsic flexors, must slacken so the dorsal interosseous can abduct the finger. This action is an example of the biomechanical system that provides balance between the muscles to let the fingers grasp. The power and strength of this grasp comes from the adductor pollicis and the thumb flexors.

Interesting Information

The thumb adductor muscle is regarded by Strickland as "perhaps the most important intrinsic muscle" (1995, p. 31). The lateral pinch is considered one of most functional grasps (Tubiana et al., 1996).

Functional Uses

This grasp can be used for inserting change or an electronic card into a machine, holding a key, putting mail into a mail slot, inserting a disc into a computer, and pulling up zippers during dressing.

PAD TO PAD GRASP

(Smith & Benge, 1985)

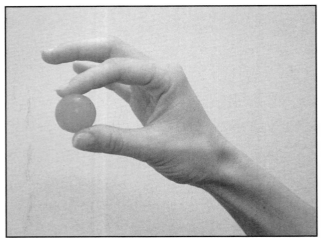

Figure 6-36. Observe that the object is secured between the pads of the finger and thumb.

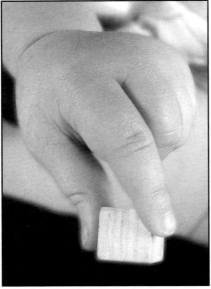

Figure 6-37. Note that the ulnar fingers may be extended for balance or flexed into the palm for greater stability.

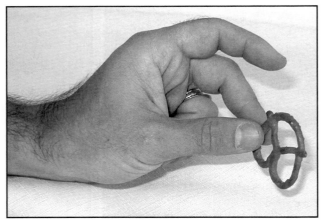

Figure 6-38. Notice that either the index or middle finger may be used to accomplish the pad to pad grasp.

Alternative Grasp Names

- *Pincer Prehension* (Castner, 1932)
- *Standard Palmar Pinch* (Weiss & Flatt, 1971)
- *Adult* (Connolly & Elliot, 1972; Connolly, 1973)
- *Inferior Pincer Grasp* (Gesell & Amatruda, 1974)
- *Tip Prehension* (Kamakura et al., 1980)
- *Adult Digital* (Moss & Hogg, 1981)
- *Two-Point Pinch* (Smith & Benge, 1985)
- *Superior Pinch* (Gilfoyle et al., 1990)
- *Pincer Grasp* (Erhardt, 1994; Duff, 1995, Exner, 2001)
- *Superior Pincer Grasp* (Case-Smith & Bigsby, 2000)

Description

This grasp is characterized by the pad of the thumb in opposition to the pad of the index or middle finger. The ulnar fingers may be extended for balance or flexed in the palm for support. Both the longitudinal arch and the transverse arches support the posture required for this grasp. The longitudinal arch assists the hand with flexion of the IP and MCP joints in this grasp and provides flexibility by flattening and cupping the palm and fingers. This flexibility allows the person to pick up objects that vary in size (Duncan, 1989). The relatively rigid transverse carpal arch provides the stability from which the distal structures can move. This grasp lacks the DIP flexion that forms the distinct "O" characteristic of the more precise tip pinch. A similar grasp is used by the developing child and appears in the developmental chapter as the pincer grasp.

Muscles

The extensor longus and brevis position the thumb in extension, while the thumb intrinsics are used to hold the object. The extrinsic flexors of the index or middle finger provide counterpressure for holding objects.

Interesting Information

Several characteristics of the skin on the pads of the fingers contribute to the success of the precision grip. One

PAD TO PAD GRASP, CONTINUED

(Smith & Benge, 1985)

factor is the highly textured surface area of the skin provided by the papillary ridges etched with fingerprints that have grooves, lines, folds and furrows, and sweat pores to provide moistness. The thumb and fingers also have a distinct fat pad and skin that is mobile. This is in contrast to the skin center of the palm, which is tightly fastened with no distinct fat pad. This padded surface of the thumb and fingers allows for increased stabilization of small objects. According to the theory of evolution, the opposable thumb, which is necessary for this type of grasp, emerged 1.75 million years ago (Napier, 1993). This grasp provides more stability when compared to the tip pinch, but is less stable than the three jaw chuck.

Functional Uses

Children and adults use this grasp to pick up finger foods or small toys, as well as to hold thread for threading a needle.

THREE JAW CHUCK

(Duff, 1995; Trombly 1995a; Exner, 2001)

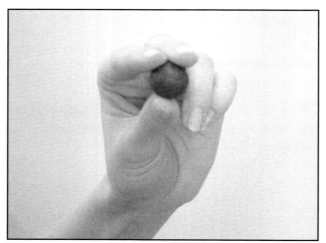

Figure 6-39. Note the full opposition of the thumb to the pads both the index and middle finger in the three jaw chuck.

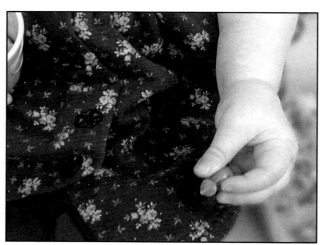

Figure 6-41. The three jaw chuck is similar to the pad to pad but the middle finger is added to secure the object being grasped.

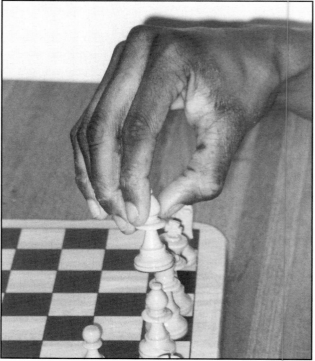

Figure 6-40. Note that the ulnar fingers may be extended for balance or flexed into the palm for greater stability.

- *Three-Jawed Chuck* (Wilson, 1998)
- *Baseball Grip* (Wilson, 1998)

Description

This grasp is characterized by the pad of the thumb in opposition to the pads of both the index and middle fingers. This combination of thumb and fingers in opposition provides a stability of prehension (Exner, 2001) and is "perhaps the most important movement of the human hand" (Napier, 1993, p. 55). As mentioned earlier, rotation of the thumb is the key element to opposition and is dependent on the saddle joint of the thumb. The flexible transverse metacarpal arch is formed slightly below or proximal to the MCP joint in this grasp. The transverse carpal arch is comprised of the distal carpal bones and is a stable point that allows a pivot for the interplay of wrist and middle finger bones during this grasp (Coppard & Lohman, 1996). The ulnar fingers may be extended for balance or flexed into the palm for support. The wrist is usually in a neutral position or slightly extended.

Alternative Grasp Names

- *Forefinger Grasp* (Halverson, 1931; Ammon & Etzel, 1977)
- *Three-Point Palmar Pinch* (Sherik et al., 1971)
- *Three-Point Pinch* (Smith & Benge, 1985)
- *3-Jawed Chuck Grasp* (Erhardt, 1994)
- *Palmar Pinch* (Trombly, 1995a)
- *Palmar Prehension* (Belkin et al., 1996)

THREE JAW CHUCK, CONTINUED

(Duff, 1995; Trombly 1995a; Exner, 2001)

Muscles

The intrinsic muscles of the thumb are very active in placing and holding the thumb in opposition. The long thumb extensor acts as antagonist to hold the IP joint in some flexion or the muscle may act as an agonist and hold the IP joint in extension. The extrinsic muscles of the index and middle fingers place the IP joints in flexion or extension as the lumbricals flex the MCP joints.

Interesting Information

This is a highly functional grasp because it positions the hand so the sensitive pads of the thumb and finger have a broad area of intimate contact, which is important for manipulation and touch. This grasp maximizes the rich sensory components of the papillary skin, which makes for effective handling of smaller objects that may also be delicate.

Developmentally, this grasp appears around 10 to 12 months of age in the typically developing child (Gesell & Amatruda, 1974; Erhardt, 1994). It then rapidly accelerates in use because it is used in many functional activities, such as picking up food and manipulating utensils for eating.

Functional Uses

The adult may use this grasp for sewing activities, eating small pieces of food, and grasping delicate objects (i.e., a flower).

TIP PINCH

(Exner, 2001)

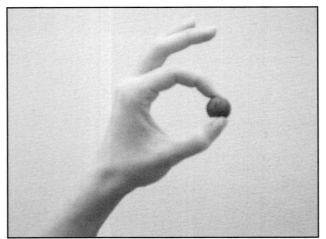

Figure 6-42. Notice the flexion of the DIP of the finger that brings the tip of the finger to the pad of the thumb and forms the distinct "O," that differentiates this grasp from the pad to pad.

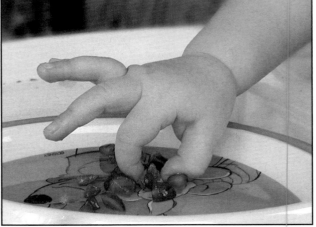

Figure 6-43. The use of the tips of the pads of the finger and thumb allow greater precision when grasping and object.

Alternative Grasp Names

- *Superior Forefinger Grasp or Superior Finger Grasp* (Halverson, 1931)
- *Neat Pincer Grasp* (Gesell & Amatruda, 1974; Ammon & Etzel, 1977; Newborg et al., 1984; Parks, 1988; Johnson-Martin et al., 1991; Provence et al., 1995)
- *Pincer Grasp* (Parks, 1988)
- *Superior Pincer Grasp* (Illingworth, 1991; Case-Smith, 1995; Duff, 1995; Bruni, 1998)
- *Prehension* (Gilfoyle et al., 1990)
- *Fine Pincher Grasp* (Erhardt, 1994)
- *Pinch* (Bruni, 1998)

Description

This grasp is exemplified by opposition of the thumb (Napier, 1993; Exner, 2001) with the tip of the index [or middle] finger so that a circle is formed (Sherik et al., 1971). According to Exner (2001) there is flexion in all joints of the finger. A similar grasp is used by the developing child and appears in the developmental chapter as the neat pincer grasp.

Muscles

The most important muscles used in this grasp are the extrinsics (for index finger flexion) and the dorsal

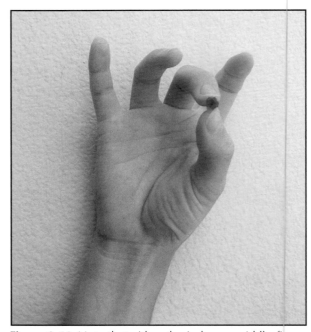

Figure 6-44. Note that either the index or middle finger can be used to accomplish the tip pinch.

interosseous. The interosseous (as well as the lumbricals) are well endowed with special nerve endings that provide a positional sense that has no equal anywhere else in the body (Napier, 1993). This position sense is especially vital in a grasp that requires such precision as the tip pinch.

TIP PINCH, CONTINUED

(Exner, 2001)

Also needed are the extrinsic thumb flexors to flex the IP joint and the intrinsics of the thumb for abduction, rotation, and opposition.

Interesting Information

Adequate length of the thumb and index finger are essential in accomplishing tip-to-pad contact in this grasp (Napier, 1993). People with genetic conditions, such as persons with Down syndrome, have short thumbs and may have difficulty with this grasp. The richly endowed tactile surfaces of the fingertips and thumb pads allow an array of sensory and somatosensory feedback. With this sensory feedback, the person adjusts the pressure of the grasp in order to hold the object. The eye-hand coordination, plus the ability to isolate the index finger and oppose the thumb, are also necessary to successfully use this grasp. The tip pinch that lacks the "O" formed by the arches, web space, and support of an intact thumb and index finger has compromised function when grasping objects (Tubiana et al., 1996). Approximately 15 muscles have a direct or indirect contribution in exerting force in order to hold a small object (Hepp-Reymond, Huesler, & Maier, 1996). Developmentally, this grasp appears at approximately 10 to 12 months of age.

Functional Uses

It is one of the most precise grasp and is used for picking up delicate, fine, or small objects. This grasp can be used for picking up and /or fastening jewelry and holding a paper clip or other small objects.

TRANSVERSE DIGITAL GRASP

(Connolly & Elliott, 1972; Moss & Hogg, 1981)

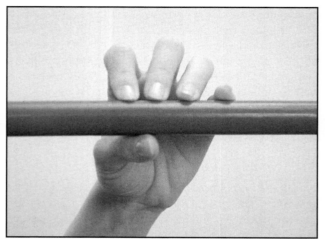

Figure 6-45. Note that the object contacts the hand only at the fingertips and thumb in this grasp.

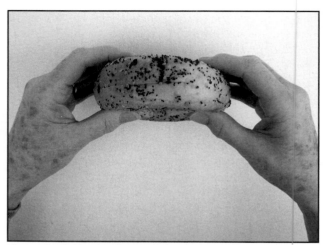

Figure 6-46. Varying finger abduction as well as MCP and IP flexion may be seen in the transverse digital grasp, depending on the size of the object.

Description

In this prehension pattern, "the object lies transversely along the fingertips and opposed by the thumb. This is a precision grip, though the range of intrinsic movements is limited to quite a small amount of lateral rotation by the fingers" (Connolly, 1973, p. 350).

Muscles

The extrinsic flexors of all the fingers flex the IP joints, and the lumbricals flex the MCP joints of all the fingers. Extrinsic muscles extend the CMC joint and flex the MCP joint of the thumb. The intrinsic muscles adduct the thumb. The extensor muscles are also important in this grasp. As stated by Bendz (1980, p. 115), "...it should be remembered that the passive tension of a motor system plays as big a role in the mutual balance of motor forces as does the system's active contraction. The passive tension is dynamic..." This biomechanical balance is necessary for functional grasps.

Interesting Information

According to the theory of evolution, the use of precision grasps evolved approximately 60,000 years ago, while power grasps have been used for approximately 3 to 4 million years (Wilson, 1998).

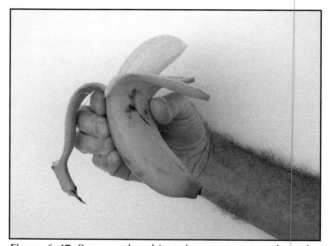

Figure 6-47. Because the object does not contact the palm in the transverse digital grasp, it is considered a precision grasp.

Functional Uses

This grasp is optimal for playing a musical instrument like a flute or clarinet, holding a candy bar, or holding a hamburger with two hands while eating it.

MISCELLANEOUS GRASPS

FUNCTIONAL SCISSORS GRASP

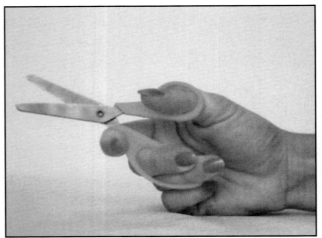

Figure 6-48. This photograph is an example in which the middle and ring fingers are held in the loop of the scissors, while the index finger guides the cutting.

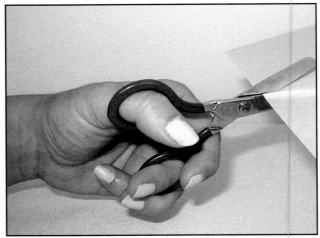

Figure 6-49. Because of the smaller size of this scissor loop, only the middle finger is placed in the loop in this photograph.

Alternative Grasp Names

*   *Power Grip-Distal Type* (Kamakura et al., 1980)
*   *Scissors Grasp* (Myers, 1992)

Description

In this grasp, the thumb and the middle finger, or both the middle and ring fingers (depending on the size of the loops) are placed in the scissor loops (Schneck & Battaglia, 1992). The finger(s) and thumb are stabilized against the loops near the DIP joints (Myers, 1992; Benbow, 1995). The index finger is placed around the bottom scissors loop to provide stability and strength as well as direct the cutting action (Schneck & Battaglia, 1992). The ulnar digits are flexed into the palm, separating the motor functions of the two sides of the hand.

Muscles

The thumb is stabilized as a "post" by the thumb extrinsic muscles. The intrinsic muscles of the thumb pro-vide the opposition, adduction, and abduction during the cutting movements. The flexor extrinsics, along with the lumbricals and interossei, flex the finger joints (Clarkson & Gilewich, 1989).

Interesting Information

Often children position the thumb and index finger in the scissors loops, but this position does not allow for skilled control of the scissors and does not assist in developing the hand for fine-motor skill (Myers, 1992). "When scissors are held incorrectly, cutting activities are performed primarily by the larger muscles of the forearm…" (Myers, 1992, p. 52). If scissors are positioned correctly and they fit a child's hand well, cutting activities develop the same intrinsic muscles that are used to manipulate a pencil in a mature tripod grasp (Myers, 1992).

Functional Uses

Scissors can be used for cutting paper, cloth, food, plants, hair, and other miscellaneous items.

HOOK GRASP

(Napier, 1956, 1993; Sherik et al., 1971; Weiss & Flatt, 1971; Exner, 2001)

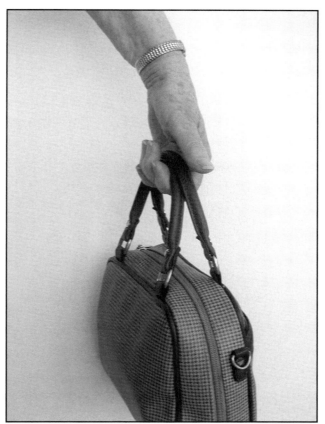

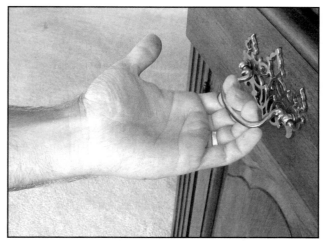

Figure 6-51. Because less power is needed to open the drawer (as compared to holding the purse), only the IP joints of the fingers flex to accomplish this task.

Figure 6-50. Note the lack of contact of the thumb and the palm while the IP and MCP joints flex to support the weight of the object.

Alternative Grasp Name

- *Power Grip-Hook Type* (Kamakura et al., 1980)

Description

This grasp uses only the fingers and does not involve the palm or the thumb. It is a "subsidiary" grasp, because it is neither a power nor precision grasp (Napier, 1993, p. 62). Characteristics of the hook grasp include adducted fingers that are flexed at the IP joints, while the transverse arch is somewhat flat (Sherik et al., 1971). Flexion of the MCP joints provides power to the grasp (Weiss & Flatt, 1971).

Muscles

The extrinsic finger flexors and extensor muscles (with stabilization of the lumbricals for flexion of the fingers' MCP joints) are important for this grasp. The thumb has no direct contact with the object in this grasp.

Interesting Information

Phylogenetically, it is a very old grasp. For millions of years and into the present, this grasp, according to the theory of evolution, was and is used for brachiation (swinging using the arms). This grasp is well-suited for our use in carrying heavy objects, such as a briefcase; however, continual use may contribute to tendonitis in the elbow.

Functional Uses

It is used to a carry a heavy suitcase and can be used while rock climbing.

INTERDIGITAL GRASP

(Moss & Hogg, 1981)

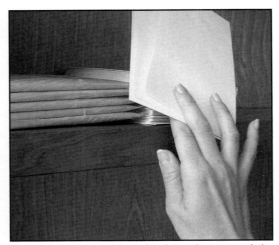

Figure 6-52. Note the lack of involvement of the thumb and palm.

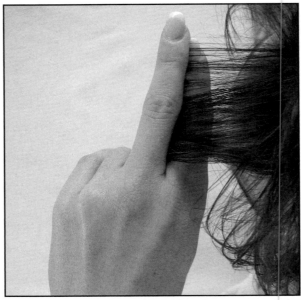

Figure 6-53. Note the variation in the position of the ulnar fingers.

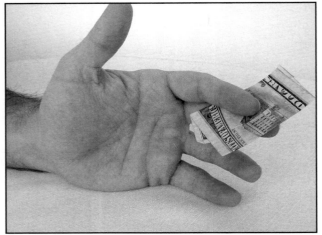

Figure 6-54. Finger adductors secure the object in the interdigital grasp.

Alternative Grasp Name

- *Adduction Grip* (Kamakura et al., 1980)

Description

This prehension pattern is characterized by the extension of the MCP and IP joints of the fingers. The object is secured by adduction of the fingers against the object. There is no thumb involvement.

Muscles

The primary movers in this prehensile grasp would be the lumbricals, and the palmar and dorsal interossei supplied by the median and ulnar nerves. Strong adductors are very important for this grasp. Stabilization of the hand and fingers comes from the extrinsic finger extensors, as well as the collateral ligaments.

Interesting Information

This grasp is representative of the type of grasps that many authors find difficult to define, organize, and analyze. This grasp is neither a power grasp, because it does not involve the palm and finger pads, nor is it a precision grasp that uses only the pads of the fingers (Napier, 1993).

Functional Uses

This grasp allows the hand to extend its reaching length by extending the fingers to grasp an object in tight or small spaces. In certain progressive neurologic diseases, such as muscular dystrophy, this grasp can be used to hold objects for grooming and utensils for eating. A person with intact muscles and nerves can use this grasp to hold a credit card or paper money, or grab a pen or pencil from a standing container.

LUMBRICAL GRASP

(Tyldesley & Grieve, 1996)

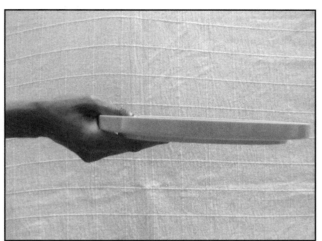

Figure 6-55. Note the entire volar aspect of the fingers and thumb can be used to secure the object and, if more power is needed, palmar contact occurs, such as in this picture of a plate. This can be contrasted with the transverse digital grasp in that only the pads of the digits are used (hence its classification as a precision grasp).

Alternative Grasp Names

- *Parallel Extension Grip* (Kamakura et al., 1980)
- *Plate Grip* (Tyldesley & Grieve, 1996)
- *Five-Jawed Cradle Grip* (Wilson, 1998)

Description

This grasp is characterized by MCP flexion and, often, IP extension of the fingers. "The thumb is opposed across the palmar surface of the fingers" (Tyldesley & Grieve, 1996, p. 171). The degree of MCP flexion varies greatly in the fingers but is greatest in the little finger (Kamakura et al., 1980). The object touches the thenar eminence of the thumb when power is needed, but no other parts of the palm are touched when using this grasp (Kamakura et al., 1980). The fingers abduct when more power is needed for grasping heavier objects.

Muscles

The intrinsic muscles of the thumb oppose or adduct and stabilize the thumb. The extrinsic muscles of the

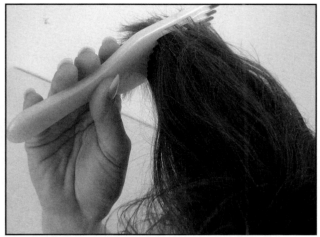

Figure 6-56. In this example of the lumbrical grasp less power is needed, so the object lies between the fingers and the thumb but does not contact the palm.

thumb provide IP extension. The fingers are held in extension at the IP joints, and are flexed at the MCP joints primarily by the lumbricals and interossei. The lumbricals are regarded as the "workhorses" of the hand, yet researchers are still unclear about their precise role (Falkenstein & Weiss-Lessard, 1999).

Interesting Information

Depending on the weight of the object and the necessary palmar contact to increase power, this grasp may be classified as a power or precision grasp. Because the MCP flexion is an essential component of most grasps, a disruption of this movement can devastate hand function. The lumbrical grasp is an example of a grasp where MCP flexion is vital.

Functional Uses

This grasp is often used when carrying items in the horizontal plane, such as a plate, saucer, or a stack of papers. It is also used when carrying books and other objects in the vertical plane.

RAKING GRASP

(Parks, 1988)

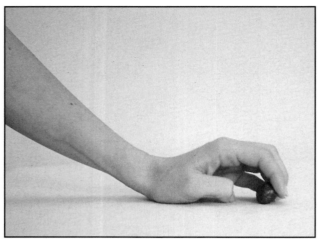

Figure 6-57. Notice that the thumb does not contact the object in this example.

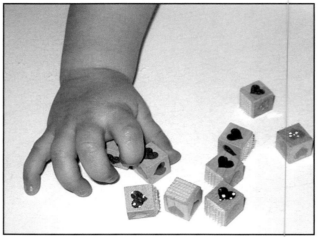

Figure 6-58. Although the thumb is in contact with the object in this example of the raking grasp, it is not active in bringing the object into the palm.

Alternative Grasp Names

- *Radial Raking* (Gesell & Amatruda, 1974)
- *Inferior Scissors Grasp* (Erhardt, 1994)
- *Crude Raking* (Exner, 2001)

Description

Raking of the object is the most characteristic feature of this grasp. This grasp, as described by Gesell and Amatruda (1974), is a child's "first attempts to pick up small items using all the fingers to 'rake' them into the palm" (Bruni, 1998, p. 65). The IP joints are flexed in all the fingers. The thumb does not actively participate in this grasp. The arches are enlisted to position the digits to rake the object. The heel of the hand on the surface is a stabilizing force. The wrist is slightly extended, and movement of the arm is necessary to provide the raking motion to grasp or move the object (Erhardt, 1994).

Muscles

The extrinsic muscles flex the IP joints of the fingers, and the lumbricals flex the MCP joints of the fingers.

Interesting Information

This grasp can be used by individuals with typically functioning hands, as well as by those individuals with weak intrinsic muscles in the thumb and fingers. Developmentally, this grasp emerges around 7 months (Parks, 1988) and appears before finger isolation has developed.

Functional Uses

Some functional uses of this grasp for adults would be to gather cards off a table; and for children, to gather small objects (ie, pellets or other toys).

NONPREHENSILE HAND MOVEMENTS

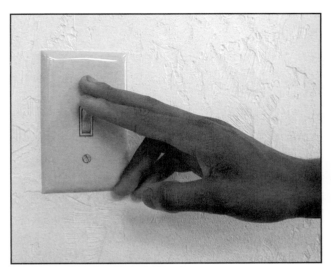

Figure 6-59. Nonprehensile hand movement.

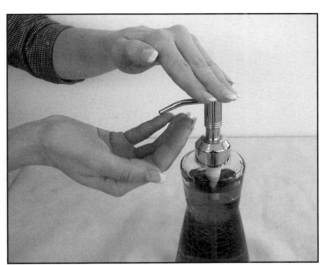

Figure 6-60. Nonprehensile hand movement.

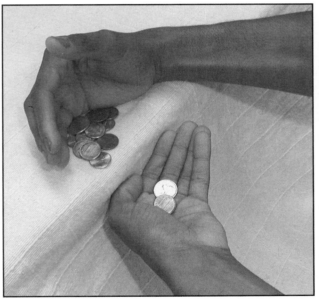

Figure 6-61. Nonprehensile hand movement.

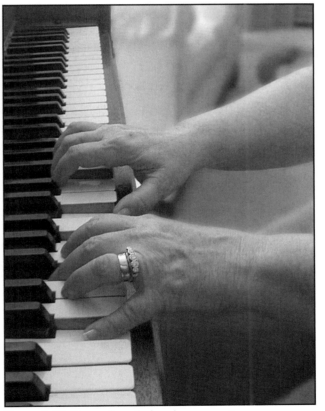

Figure 6-62. Nonprehensile hand movement.

Hand movements can be separated into two distinct groups: prehensile and nonprehensile. Prehensile movements are movements in which "an object is seized and held partly or wholly within the compass of the hand" (Napier, 1956). These include the grasps discussed earlier in this chapter.

In contrast, nonprehensile movements are those in which "movements are accomplished by pushing or lifting the object with the fingers or the entire hand" (Exner, 2001 p. 294). The pictures illustrate how nonprehensile hand movements are used in daily functional activities.

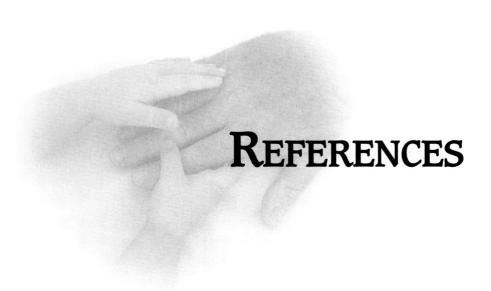

REFERENCES

Ammon, J. E., & Etzel, M. E. (1977). Sensorimotor organization in reach and prehension: A developmental model. *Phys Ther, 57,* 7-14.

Amundson, S. J. (1995). *Evaluation of children's handwriting ETCH Examiner's manual.* Homer, AK: O. T. KIDS.

Amundson, S. J. (1998). *Tricks for written communication techniques for rebuilding and improving children's school skills.* Homer, AK: O. T. KIDS.

Ayres, A. J. (1954). Ontogenetic principles in the development of arm and hand functions. *Am J Occup Ther, 8,* 95-99.

Barnes, M. R., Crutchfield, C. A., & Heriza, C. B. (1978). *The neurophysiological basis of patient treatment* (Vol. 2). Morgantown, WV: Stokesville Publishing.

Bell, C. (1834). *The hand, its mechanism and vital endowments, as evincing design: The Bridgewater treatise on the power, wisdom, and goodness of God as manifested in the creation.* (Treatise IV.) New York: Harper and Brothers.

Bell-Krotoski, J., Weinstein, S., & Weinstein, C. (1993). Testing sensibility, including touch-pressure, two-point discrimination, point localization, and vibration. *J Hand Ther, 2,* 114-123.

Belkin, J., English, C. B., Adler, C., & Pedretti, L. (1996). Orthotics. In L.W. Pedretti (Ed.), *Occupational therapy practice skills for physical dysfunction* (4th ed., pp. 319-349). St. Louis, MO: Mosby-Year Book.

Benbow, M. (1995). Principles and practices of handwriting. In A. Henderson & C. Pehoski (Eds.), *Hand function in the child* (pp. 255-281). St. Louis, MO: Mosby-Year Book.

Benbow, M. (1999). *Fine motor development activities to develop hand skills in young children.* Columbus, OH: Zaner-Bloser

Benbow, M. (2002). Hand skills and handwriting. In S. A. Cermak & D. Larkin (eds.), *Developmental coordination disorder* (pp. 248-279). Australia: Delmar.

Bendz, P. (1980). The motor balance of the fingers of the open hand. Scand J *Rehabil Med, 12,* 115-121.

Bergmann, K. P. (1990). Incidence of atypical pencil grasps among nondysfunctional adults. *Am J Occup Ther, 44,* 736-740.

Boehme, R. (1988). *Improving upper body control.* Tucson, AZ: Therapy Skill Builders.

Brandenburg, M. A., Hawkins, L., & Quick, G. (1999). Hand injuries. Part 1: Initial evaluation and wound care. *Consultant, 39,* 3226-3243.

Bruni, M. (1998). *Fine motor skills in children with Down syndrome: A guide for parents and professionals.* Bethesda MD: Woodbine House.

Buckland, D., McCoy, J., & Edwards, S. (1999). *The hand function process in self-care activities.* Unpublished master's project, Western Michigan University, Kalamazoo, MI.

Callinan, N. (2002). Construction of hand splints. In C. A. Trombly & M. V. Radomski (Eds.), *Occupational therapy for physical dysfunction* (5th ed., pp. 351-370). Philadelphia: Lippincott, Williams & Wilkins.

Capener, N. (1956). The hand in surgery. *J Bone Joint Am, 38B(1),* 128-140.

Case-Smith, J. (1995). Grasp release and bimanual skills in the first two years of life. In A. Henderson & C. Pehoski (Eds.), *Hand function in the child* (pp. 113-135). St. Louis, MO: Mosby-Year Book.

Case-Smith, J. (2002). Effectiveness of school-based occupational therapy intervention of handwriting. *Am J Occup Ther, 56,* 17-25.

Case-Smith, J., & Bigsby, R. (2000). *Posture and fine motor assessment in infants.* Tucson, AZ: Therapy Skill Builders.

Castner, B. M. (1932). The development of fine prehension in infancy. *Genetic Psychology Monographs, 12,* 105-193.

Clarkson, H. M., & Gilewich, G. B. (1989). *Musculoskeletal assessment joint range of motion and manual muscle strength.* Baltimore, MD: Williams & Wilkins.

Conner, F. P., Williamson, G. G., & Siepp, J. M. (1978). *Program guide for infants and toddlers with neurological and other developmental disabilities.* New York: Teachers College Press.

Connolly, K. (1973). Factors influencing the learning of manual skills by young children. In R. A. Hinde & J. Stevenson-Hinde (Eds.), *Constraints on learning* (pp. 337-363). London: Academic Press.

Connolly, K., & Elliott, J. (1972). The evolution and ontogeny of hand function. In N. Blurton Jones (Ed.), *Ethological studies of child behavior.* Cambridge, UK: Cambridge University Press.

Cooper, C. (2002). Hand impairments. In C. A. Trombly & M. V. Radomski (Eds.), *Occupational therapy for physical dysfunction* (5th ed., pp. 927-963). Philadelphia: Lippincott, Williams & Wilkins

Coppard, B. M., & Lohman, H. (1996). *Introduction to splinting: A critical-thinking and problem solving approach.* St. Louis, MO: Mosby-Year Book.

Corbetta, D., & Mounoud, P. (1990). Early development of grasping and manipulation. In C. Bard, M. Fleury, & L. Hay (Eds.), *Development of eye-hand coordination across the life span* (pp. 188-213). Columbia, SC: University of South Carolina.

Dellon, A., & Kallman C. (1983). Evaluation of functional sensation in the hand. *J Hand Surg, 8,* 865-870.

Dennis, J. L., & Swinth, Y. (2001). Pencil grasp and children's handwriting legibility during different-length writing tasks. *Am J Occup Ther, 55,* 175-183.

Duff, S. V. (1995). Prehension. In D. Cech & S. T. Martin (Eds.), *Functional movement development across the life span* (pp. 313-353). Philadelphia: W. B. Saunders.

Duff, S., Shumway-Cook, A., & Woollacott, M. H. (2001). Clinical management of the patient with reach, grasp, and manipulation disorders. In A. Shumway-Cook, & M. H. Woollacott (Eds.), *Motor control theory and practical applications* (2nd ed). Philadelphia: Lippincott Williams & Wilkins.

Duncan, R. (1989). Basic principles of splinting the hand. *Phys Ther, 69,* 1104-1113.

Edwards, S. J., & Lafreniere, M. K. (1995). Hand function in the Down syndrome population. In A. Henderson & C. Pehoski (Eds.), *Hand function in the child* (pp. 299-311). St. Louis, MO: Mosby-Year Book.

Elliott, J. M., & Connolly, K. J. (1984). A classification of manipulative hand movements. *Dev Med Child Neurol, 26,* 283-296.

Erhardt, R. P. (1992). Eye-hand coordination. In J. Case-Smith & C. Pehoski (Eds.), *Development of hand skills in the child.* (pp. 13-33). Bethesda, MD: American Occupational Therapy Association.

Erhardt, R. P. (1994). *Developmental hand dysfunction theory assessment and treatment.* Tucson, AZ: Therapy Skill Builders.

Exner, C. E. (2001). Development of hand skills. In J. Case-Smith (Ed.), *Occupational therapy for children* (4th ed., pp. 289-328). St. Louis, MO: Mosby-Year Book.

Falkenstein, N., & Weiss-Lessard, S. (1999). *Hand rehabilitation a quick reference guide and review.* St. Louis, MO: Mosby-Year Book.

Fiorentino, M. R. (1973). *Reflex testing methods for evaluating CNS development* (2nd ed.). Springfield, IL: Bannerstone House.

Fiorentino, M. R. (1981). *A basis for sensorimotor development—Normal and abnormal.* Springfield, IL: Bannerstone House.

Flatt, A. E. (1972). Restoration of rheumatoid finger joint function III. *J Bone Joint Surg Am, 54A,* 1317-1322.

Gesell, A. L., & Amatruda, C. S. (1974). In H. Knobloch, & B. Pasamanick (Eds.), *Gesell and Amatruda's developmental diagnosis: The evaluation and management of normal and abnormal neuropsychologic development in infancy and childhood* (3rd ed.). Hagerstown, MD: Harper & Row Publishers.

Gilfoyle, E. M., Grady, A. P., & Moore, J. C. (1990). *Children adapt* (2nd ed.). Thorofare, NJ: SLACK Incorporated.

Goodgold, S. A. (1983). Handwriting movement quality in prekindergarten and kindergarten children. *Arch Phys Med Rehabil, 64,* 471-475.

Gordon, A. M., & Duff, S. V. (1999). Relationships between clinical measures and fine manipulative control in children with hemiplegic cerebral palsy. *Dev Med Child Neurol, 41,* 586-591

Halverson, H. M. (1931). An experimental study of prehension in infants by means of systematic cinema records. *Genetic Psychology Monographs, 10,* 107-286.

Halverson, H. M., Thompson, H., Ilg, F. L., Castner, B. M., Ames, L. B., Gesell, A., et al. (1940). *The first five years of life: A guide to the study of preschool children.* New York: Harper & Brothers Publishers.

Hanft, B., & Marsh, D. (1993). *Getting a grip on handwriting: A self-guided video and manual.* Rockville, MD: American Occupational Therapy Association.

Hazelton, F. T., Smidt, G. L., Flatt, A. E., & Stephens, R. I. (1975). The influence of wrist position on the force produced by the finger flexors. *J Biomech, 8,* 301-306.

Henderson, A., & Pehoski, C. (Eds.) (1995). *Hand function in the child.* St. Louis, MO: Mosby-Year Book.

Hepp-Reymond, M. C., Huesler, E. J., & Maier, M. A. (1996). Precision grip in humans. In A. M. Wing, P. Haggard, & J. R. Flanagan (Eds.), Hand and brain: The neurophysiology and psychology of hand movements (pp. 37-62). San Diego, CA: Academic Press.

Hirschel, A., Pehoski, C., & Coryell, J. (1990). Environmental support and the development of grasp in infants. Am J Occup Ther, 44, 721-727.

Hislop, H. J., & Montgomery, J. (1995). Daniels and Worthingham's muscle testing. Philadelphia: W. B. Saunders.

Hogg, J., & Moss, S. C. (1983). Prehensile development in Down syndrome. British Journal of Developmental Psychology, 1, 189-204.

Illingworth, R. S. (1963). The development of the infant and young child: Normal and abnormal. London: E & S Livingstone.

Illingworth, R. S. (1991). The normal child: Some problems of the early years and their treatment (10th ed.). Edinburgh: Churchill-Livingstone.

Jacobson, C., & Sperling, L. (1976). Classification of the hand-grip. J Occup Med, 18, 395-398.

Johnson-Martin, N. M., Jens, K. G., Attermeier, S. M., & Hacker, B. J. (1991). The Carolina curriculum for infants and toddlers with special needs (2nd ed.). Baltimore, MD: Paul H. Brookes Publishing.

Kamakura, N., Matsuo, M., Ishii, H., Mitsuboshi, F., & Miura, Y. (1980). Patterns of static prehension in normal hands. Am J Occup Ther, 34, 437-445.

Link, L., Lukens, S., & Bush, M. A. (1995). Spherical grip strength in children 3 to 6 years old. Am J Occup Ther, 33, 318-326.

Lockhart, R. D., Hamilton, G. F., & Fyfe, F. W. (1959). Anatomy of the human body. Philadelphia: J. B. Lippincott.

Long, C., Conrad, P. W., Hall, E. A., & Furler, S. L. (1970). Intrinsic-extrinsic muscle control of the hand in power and precision handling. J Bone Joint Surg Am, 52A, 853-867.

McBride, E. D. (1942). Disability evaluation: Principles of treatment of compensable injuries (2nd ed.). Philadelphia: J. B. Lippincott.

Morrison, A. (1978). Occupational therapy for writing difficulties in spina bifida children with myelomeningocele and hydrocephalus. British Journal of Occupational Therapy, 40, 394-398.

Moss, S. C., & Hogg, J. (1981). Development of hand function in mentally handicapped and nonhandicapped preschool children. In P. Mittler (Ed.), Frontiers of knowledge in mental retardation. Social, educational, and behavioral aspects (Vol. 1, pp. 35-44). Baltimore, MD: University Park Press.

Murray, E. A. (1995). Hand preference and its development. In A. Henderson, & C. Pehoski (Eds.), Hand function in the child (pp. 154-163). St. Louis, MO: Mosby-Year Book.

Myers, C. A. (1992). Therapeutic fine-motor activities for preschoolers. In J. Case-Smith, & C. Pehoski (Eds.), Development of hand skills in the child (pp. 47-61). Bethesda, MD: American Occupational Therapy Association.

Nakada, M., & Uchida, H. (1997). Case study of a five-stage sensory reeducation program. Hand Therapy, 10, 232-239.

Napier, J. R. (1956). The prehensile movements of the human hand. J Bone Joint Surg Am, 39B(4), 902-913.

Napier, J. R. (1993). Hands (Rev. ed.). Princeton, NJ: Princeton University Press.

Newborg, J., Stock, J. R., Wnek, L., Guidubaldi, J., & Suinicki, J. (1984). Battelle developmental inventory. Allen, TX: DLM Teaching Resources.

Otto, W., Rarick, G. L., Armstrong, J., & Koepke, M. (1966). Evaluation of modified grip in handwriting. Perceptual and Motor Skills, 22, 310.

Pact, V., Sirotkin-Roses, M., & Beatus, J. (1984). The muscle testing handbook. Boston, MA: Little, Brown, and Company.

Parks, S. (Ed.). (1988). Help...at home. Palo Alto, CA: VORT.

Pehoski, C. (1992). Central nervous system control of precision movements of the hand. In J. Case-Smith, & C. Pehoski (Eds.), Development of hand skills in the child (pp.1-11). Bethesda, MD: American Occupational Therapy Association.

Penso, D. E. (1990). Keyboard, graphic, and handwriting skills: Helping people with motor disabilities. London: Chapman and Hall.

Peterson, C. Q. (1999). The effect of an occupational therapy intervention on handwriting in academically at-risk first graders. UMI Dissertation Services, No. 9946543.

Philips, C. A. (1995). Impairments of hand function. In C. A. Trombly (Ed.), Occupational therapy for physical dysfunction (4th ed., pp. 773-794). Baltimore, MD: Williams and Wilkins.

Provence, S., Erikson, J., Vater, S., & Palmeri, S. (1995). Infant-toddler developmental assessment. Chicago: Riverside Publishing.

Reed, K. L. (1991). Quick reference to occupational therapy. Gaithersburg, MD: Aspen Publishers.

Rosenbloom, L., & Horton, M. E. (1971). The maturation of fine prehension in young children. Dev Med Child Neurol, 13, 3-8.

Saida, Y., & Miyashita, M. (1979). Development of fine motor skill in children: Manipulation of a pencil in young children aged 2 to 6 years old. Journal of Human Movement Studies, 5, 104-113.

Sassoon, R., Nimmo-Smith, I., & Wing, A. M. (1986). An analysis of children's penholds. In H. S. R. Kao, G. P. van Galen, & R. Hoosain (Eds.), Graphonomics: Contemporary research in handwriting (pp. 93-106). Amsterdam: North Holland Press.

Schneck, C. M. (1991). Comparison of pencil grip patterns in first graders with good and poor writing skills. Am J Occup Ther, 45, 701-706.

Schneck, C., & Battaglia, C. (1992). Developing scissors skills in young children. In J. Case-Smith, & C. Pehoski (Eds.), Development of hand skills in the child (pp.79-89). Bethesda, MD: American Occupational Therapy Association.

Schneck, C. M., & Henderson, A. (1990). Descriptive analysis of the developmental progression of grip position for pencil and crayon control in nondysfunctional children. Am J Occup Ther, 44, 893-900.

Sherik, S. K., Weiss, M. W., & Flatt, A. E. (1971). Functional evaluation of congenital hand anomalies. *Am J Occup Ther, 25,* 98-104.

Simon, C. J., & Daub, M. M. (1993). Human development across the life span. In H. L. Hopkins, & H. D. Smith (Eds.), *Willard and Spackman's occupational therapy* (8th ed., pp. 95-130). Philadelphia: J. B. Lippincott.

Smith, R. O., & Benge, M. W. (1985). Pinch and grasp strength: Standardization of terminology and protocol. *Am J Occup Ther, 39,* 531-535.

Strickland, J. W. (1995). Anatomy and kinesiology of the hand. In A. Henderson, & C. Pehoski (Eds.), *Hand function in the child* (pp. 16-39). St. Louis, MO: Mosby-Year Book.

Summers, J. (2001). Joint laxity in the index finger and thumb and ts relationship to pencil grasps used by children. *Australian Occupational Therapy Journal, 48,* 132-141.

Thomine, J. M. (1981). The clinical examination of the hand. In R. Tubiana (Ed.), *The hand* (Vol. I, pp. 618-647). Philadelphia: W. B. Saunders.

Touwen, B. C. L. (1971). A study on the development of some motor phenomena in infancy. *Dev Med Child Neurol, 13,* 435-446.

Trombly, C. A. (1995a). Evaluation of biomechanical and physiological aspects of motor performance. In C. Trombly (Ed.), *Occupational therapy for physical dysfunction* (4th ed., pp. 73-156). Baltimore, MD: Williams & Wilkins.

Trombly, C. A. (1995b). Theoretical foundations for practice. In C. Trombly (Ed.), *Occupational therapy for physical dysfunction* (4th ed., pp. 15-28). Baltimore, MD: Williams & Wilkins.

Tubiana, R., Thomine, J. M., & Mackin, E. (1996). *Examination of the hand and wrist.* St. Louis, MO: Mosby-Year Book.

Twitchell, T. E. (1965a). Attitudinal reflexes. *Journal of the American Physical Therapy Association, 45,* 411-418.

Twitchell, T. E. (1965b). The automatic grasping responses of infants. *Neuropsychologia, 3,* 247-259.

Twitchell, T. E. (1965c). Normal motor development. *Journal of the American Physical Therapy Association, 45,* 419-423.

Twitchell, T. E. (1970). Reflex mechanisms and the development of prehension. In K. Connolly (Ed.), *Mechanisms of motor skills development.* London: Academic Press.

Tyldesley, B., & Grieve, J. I. (1996). *Muscles, nerves, and movement kinesiology in daily living* (2nd ed.). Oxford, UK: Blackwell Science.

University of Kansas Medical Center. (1997). *Hand kinesiology.* Retrieved February 20, 2002, from http://www2.kumc.edu/instruction/sah/handkines/kines2.html.

Van Deusen, J., & Brunt, D. (1997). *Assessment in occupational therapy and physical therapy.* Philadelphia: W. B. Saunders.

VanSant, A. F. (1994). Motor development. In J. S. Tecklin (Ed.), *Pediatric physical therapy* (2nd ed., pp. 1-22). Philadelphia: J. B. Lippincott.

Weiss, M. W., & Flatt, A. E. (1971). Functional evaluation of the congenitally anomalous hand. *Am J Occup Ther, 25,* 139-143.

Wells, K. F., & Luttgens, K. (1976). *Kinesiology: The scientific basis of human motion* (6th ed.). Philadelphia: W. B. Saunders.

Wilson, F. R. (1998). *The hand: How its use shapes the brain, language, and human culture.* New York: Pantheon Books.

Wynn-Parry, C. B. (1966). *Rehabilitation of the hand* (2nd ed.). London: Butterworth.

Ziviani, J. (1982). Children's prehension while writing: A pilot investigation. *British Journal of Occupational Therapy, 45,* 306-307.

Ziviani, J. (1983). Qualitative changes in dynamic tripod grip between seven and 14 years of age. *Dev Med Child Neurol, 25,* 778-782.

Ziviani, J., & Elkins, J. (1986). Effect of pencil grip on handwriting speed and legibility. *Educational Review, 38,* 247-257.

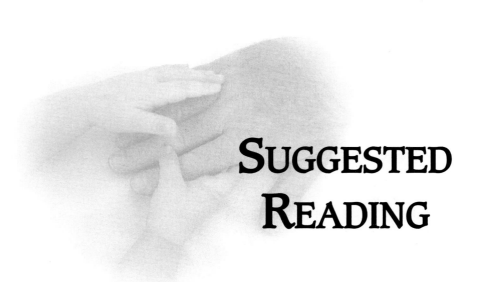

SUGGESTED READING

Alexander, R., Boehme, R., & Cupps, B. (1993). *Normal development of functional motor skills*. Tucson, AZ: Therapy Skill Builders.

Basmajian, J. V., & De Luca, C. J. (1985). *Muscles alive: Their functions revealed by electromyography* (5th ed.). Baltimore, MD: Williams & Wilkins.

Benbow, M. (2000). *Hand function and handwriting*. Rocky Mount, NC: Advanced Rehabilitation Institutes.

Cailliet, R. (1982). *Hand pain and impairment* (3rd ed.). Philadelphia: F. A. Davis Company.

Callewaert, H. (1963). For easy and legible handwriting. In V. E. Herrick (Ed.), *New horizons for research in handwriting* (pp. 39-52). Madison, WI: University of Wisconsin Press.

Coley, I. L. (1978). *Pediatric assessment of self-care activities*. St. Louis, MO: C. V. Mosby Company.

Connolly, K., & Dalgleish, M. (1989). The emergence of a tool using skill in infancy. *Developmental Psychology, 25*, 894-912.

Cunningham Amundson, S. J. (1992). Handwriting: Evaluation and intervention in school settings. In J. Case-Smith, & C. Pehoski (Eds.), *Development of hand skills in the child* (pp. 63-78). Bethesda, MD: American Occupational Therapy Association, Inc.

Dargassies, S. (1977). *Neurological development in the full term and premature neonate*. New York: Excerpta Media.

Duchenne G. (1948). *Physiology of motion* (E. Kaplan, Trans & Ed.). Philadelphia: J.B. Lippincott Company. (Original work published 1867)

Dunn, W., & Campbell, P. H. (1991). Designing pediatric service provision. In W. Dunn (Ed.), *Pediatric occupational therapy facilitating effective service provision* (pp. 139-160). Thorofare, NJ: SLACK Incorporated.

Easton, T. A. (1972). On the normal use of reflexes. *American Scientist, 60*, 591-599.

Ellis, T. S. (1878). The position of rest in fatigue and in pain. *BMJ, i*, 84.

Erhardt, R. P. (1974). Sequential levels in development of prehension. *Am J Occup Ther, 28*, 592-596.

Fenson, L., Kagan, J., Kearsley, R. B., & Zelazo, P. R. (1976). The developmental progression of manipulative play in the first two years. *Child Dev, 47*, 232-236.

Fiorentino, M. R. (1972). *Normal and abnormal development: The influence of primitive reflexes on motor development*. Springfield, IL: Bannerstone House.

Folio, M. R., & Fewell, R. R. (1983). *Peabody developmental motor scales and activity cards*. Chicago: Riverside Publishing Company.

Frankenburg, W. K., Dodds, J., Archer, P., Bresnick, B., Maschka, P., Edelman, N., et al. (1967). *Denver II training manual* (2nd ed.). Denver, CO: Denver Developmental Materials Incorporated.

Fuller, Y., & Trombly, C. A. (1997). Effects of object characteristics on female grasp patterns. *Am J Occup Ther, 51*, 481-487.

Gesell, A., Halverson, H. M., Thompson, H., Ilg, F. L., Castner, B. M., Ames, L. B., et al. (1940). *The first five years of life*. New York: Harper & Brothers.

Goldstein, K., Landis, C., Hunt, W. A., & Clarke, F. M. (1938). Moro reflex and startle pattern. *Archives of Neurology and Psychiatry, 40*, 322-327.

Hohlstein, R. R. (1982). The development of prehension in normal infants. *Am J Occup Ther, 36*, 170-176.

Humphry, R., Jewell, K., & Rosenberger, R. C. (1995). Development of in-hand manipulation and relationship with activities. *Am J Occup Ther, 49*, 763-771.

Kapandji, I. A. (1982). *The physiology of the joints: Annotated diagrams of the mechanics of the human joints* (Vol. 1, 5th ed.) (L. H. Honore, Trans.). Edinburgh, UK: Churchill Living-stone.

Kapit, W., & Elson, L. M. (1993). *The anatomy coloring book* (2nd ed.). New York: Addison-Wesley Educational Publishers, Inc.

Keogh, J., & Sugden, D. (1985). *Movement skill development*. New York: Macmillan.

Landsmeer, J. M. F. (1962). Power grip and precision handling. *Ann Rheum Dis, 21*, 164-170.

Laszlo, J. I., & Bairstow, P. J. (1984). Handwriting: Difficulties and possible solutions. *School Psychology International, 5*, 207-213.

Levine, M. D., Oberklaid, F., & Meltzer, L. (1981). Developmental output failure: A study of low productivity in school-aged children. *Pediatrics, 67*, 18-25.

Lehmkuhl, L. D., & Smith, L. K. (1983). *Brunnstrom's clinical kinesiology* (4th ed.). Philadephia: F. A. Davis Company.

McDonnell, P. M. (1979). Patterns of eye-hand coordination in the first year of life. *Canadian Journal of Psychology, 33*, 253-267.

McKale, K., & Cermak, S. A. (1992). Fine motor activities in elementary school: Preliminary findings and provisional implications for children with fine motor problems. *Am J Occup Ther, 46*, 898-903.

Napier, J. R. (1955). The form and function of the carpometacarpal joint of the thumb. *J Anat, 89*, 362-369.

Norkin, C., & Levangie, P. (1983). *Joint structure and function: A comprehensive analysis*. Philadelphia: F. A. Davis Company.

Palisano, R. J. (1988). Motor Development. In M. A. Short-DeGraff (Ed.), *Human development for occupational and physical therapists*. Baltimore, MD: Williams & Wilkins.

Paquette, L. (1998). Hand therapy: Incorporating activities into hand therapy practice. *OT Practice, 3*(6), 28-30.

Reiner, M. (1991). *The illustrated hand*. St. Paul, MN: Hand Rehabilitation, Inc.

Rochat, P. (1989). Object manipulation and exploration in 2 to 5 month old infants. *Developmental Psychology, 25*, 871-884.

Ruff, H. A. (1984). Infant's manipulative exploration of objects: Effects of age and object characteristics. *Developmental Psychology, 20*, 9-20.

Ruff, H. A., McCarton, C., Kurtzberg, D., & Vaughan, H. G., Jr. (1984). Preterm infants' manipulative exploration of objects. *Child Dev, 55*, 1166-1173.

Schieber, M. H. (1996). Individuated finger movements rejecting the labeled line hypothesis. In A. M. Wing, P. Haggard, & J. R. Flanagan (Eds.), *Hand and brain: The neurophysiology and psychology of hand movements* (pp. 81-96). San Diego, CA: Academic Press.

Semmes J., & Weinstein, S. (1960). *Somatosensory changes after penetrating brain wounds in man*. Cambridge, UK: Harvard University Press.

Seyffarth, H., & Denny-Brown, D. (1948). The grasp reflex and the instinctive grasp reaction. *Brain, 71*, 110-183.

Shumway-Cook, A., & Woollacott, M. H. (2001). *Motor control: Theory and practical applications* (2nd ed.). Philadelphia: Lippencott Williams & Wilkins.

Slocum, D. B., & Pratt, D. R. (1946). Disability evaluation for the hand. *J Bone Joint Surg Am, 28*, 491-495.

Soderberg, G. L. (1986). *Kinesiology: Application to pathological motion*. Baltimore, MD: Williams and Wilkins.

Sperling, L., & Jacobson-Sollerman, C. (1977). The grip of the healthy hand during eating. *Scand J Rehabil Med, 9*, 115-121.

Tubiana, R. (1981). *The hand* (Vol. I). Philadelphia: W. B. Saunders.

Twitchell, T. E. (1965). Variations and abnormalities of motor development. *Journal of the American Physical Therapy Association, 45*, 424-430.

van Blankenstein, M., Welbergen, U. R., & de Haas, F. H. (1962). *Le de'veloppement du nourisson*. Paris: Presses Universitaires De France.

Van Deusen, J., & Brunt, D. (1997). *Assessment in occupational therapy and physical therapy*. Philadelphia: W. B. Saunders Company.

Walsh, W. W., Belding, N. N., Taylor, E., & Nunley, J. A. (1993). The effect of upper extremity trauma on handedness. *Am J Occup Ther, 47*, 787-795.

Weiss, M. W., & Flatt, A. E. (1971). A pilot study of 198 normal children: Pinch strength and hand size in the growing hand. *Am J Occup Ther, 25*, 10-12.

Ziviani, J., & Elkins, J. (1984). An evaluation of handwriting performance. *Educational Review, 36*, 249-261.

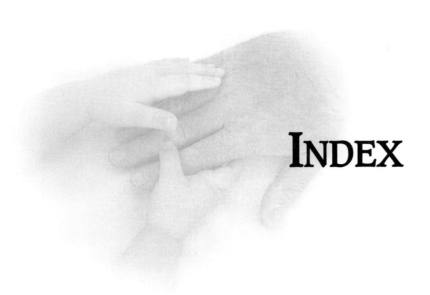

INDEX

power grasps, 87, 92-101. *See also* diagonal volar grasp
power grip-distal type. *See* functional scissors grasp
power grip-hook type. *See* hook grasp
power grip-standard type. *See* hammer grasp
pre-pincer grasp. *See* developmental scissors grasp
precision grasps, 88, 106-118
precision grip. *See* dynamic tripod grasp
prehension. *See* neat pincer grasp; tip pinch grasp
primitive grasps, 58, 64-68
primitive handwriting grasps, 61
primitive squeeze grasp. *See* crude palmar grasp; reflex squeeze grasp
pronate method. *See* digital pronate grasp
proprioception, 7
proximal palmar crease, 13
purposeful grasp, 41

quadrupod grasp, 70. *See also* dynamic quadrupod grasp

radial artery, 3
radial cross palmar grasp, 59-60, 61, 64
radial digital grasp, 42-44, 45, 51
radial nerve, 7-8
radial palmar grasp, 42-44, 45, 49. *See also* digital pronate grasp
radial raking grasp. *See* raking grasp
radiocarpal ligaments, 4
radiological exams, 1
raking grasp, 42-44, 45, 50, 86, 89, 124
reflex squeeze grasp, 42-44, 45, 46
reflexive behaviors
    definition, 31-34
reverse transverse palmar grasp, 81-82, 87, 98-99
ring grasp, 81-82, 87, 100

scars, assessment, 2-3
scissors closure grasp. *See* developmental scissors grasp
scissors grasp. *See* developmental scissors grasp; functional scissors grasp
Semmes-Weinstein monofilaments, 7
sensory discrimination tests, 7
sensory position tests, 7
skin, assessment, 2-3
spherical grasp, 81-82, 87, 101
squeeze grasp. *See* crude palmar grasp
standard palmar pinch grasp. *See* pad to pad grasp
static quadrupod grasp, 70
static quadrupod grasp, 59-60, 61
static tripod grasp, 59-60, 61, 72
static tripod posture. *See* static tripod grasp
stereognosis, 7
styloid process, 13
superior forefinger grasp. *See* neat pincer grasp; tip pinch grasp

superior palm grasp. *See* radial palmar grasp
superior pincer grasp. *See* neat pincer grasp; pad to pad grasp; pincer grasp; tip pinch grasp
superior pinch grasp. *See* pad to pad grasp; pincer grasp
surrounding mild flexion grip. *See* spherical grasp

thenar eminence, 13
thermographic exams, 1
three fingers grasp. *See* dynamic tripod grasp
three-jaw chuck grasp, 42-44, 45, 54, 83-85, 88, 114-115
three-point palmar pinch. *See* dynamic tripod grasp; three-jaw chuck grasp
thumb-finger grasp. *See* dynamic tripod grasp
tip pinch grasp, 83-85, 88, 116-117. *See* neat pincer grasp
tip prehension grasp. *See* pad to pad grasp
touch pressure sensitivity, 7
traction response, 33, 34, 36
transitional grasps, 58, 70-72
transitional handwriting grasps, 61
transverse arches, 6
transverse digital grasp, 83-85, 88, 118
transverse palmar grasp. *See* cylindrical grasp
tripod grasp. *See* radial digital grasp
tripod grip. *See* dynamic tripod grasp
tripod posture. *See* static tripod grasp
tripod variation I grasp. *See* dynamic lateral tripod grasp
Turner's syndrome, 3
two-point pinch grasp. *See* pad to pad grasp

ulnar artery, 3
ulnar nerve, assessment, 9-10
ulnar palmar grasp. *See* crude palmar grasp
ulnocarpal ligaments, 4
upper extremity, strength, 1, 41

vascular system, assessment, 3-4
ventral grasp, 80, 87, 104
volar ligaments, 5
voluntary grasp, 32
voluntary palmar grasp. *See* crude palmar grasp

web spaces, 13
whole-hand closure. *See* crude palmar grasp
whole-hand grasp. *See* developmental scissors grasp
wrist
    bones
        dorsal view, 16-17
    landmarks, 11-12
    ligaments, 18-19
    surface anatomy, 14
writing grip. *See* dynamic tripod grasp

9/12/2003